Active Management of Labour

The Dublin Experience

Active Management of Labour

The Dublin Experience

By Kieran O'Driscoll
and Declan Meagher

Department of Obstetrics and Gynaecology,
University College Dublin

Second Edition

Baillière Tindall London Philadelphia Toronto
Sydney Tokyo

Baillière Tindal
W. B. Saunders

24–28 Oval Road,
London NW1 7DX

The Curtis Center, Independence Square West
Philadelphia, PA 19106-3399, USA

1 Goldthorne Avenue
Toronto, Ontario M8Z 5T9, Canada

Harcourt Brace Jovanovich, (Australia) Pty Ltd.,
32–52 Smidmore Street, Marrickville, NSW 2204, Australia

First published 1980
Second edition 1986
Reprinted 1989

Printed and bound in Great Britain at the
University Press, Cambridge

British Library Cataloguing in Publication Data

O'Driscoll, Kieran
    Active management of labour: the Dublin
    experience.——2nd ed.
    1. Labor (Obstetrics)
    I. Title   II. Meagher, Declan
    618.4   RG651

ISBN 0-7020-1159-2

Contents

CONTENTS

SECTION III: Clinical Data

Preface

The Second Edition continues to reflect current practice in a busy obstetric service with extensive teaching commitments. Indeed, the introduction of students of various disciplines to a constructive attitude towards the birth process remains a primary objective. With regard to education generally, there has been steady progress towards the ideal of an integrated system that takes cognizance of expectant mothers also. During the time since the First Edition, the subject of caesarean section rates has come to be widely acknowledged as a medical issue with far-reaching social implications; searching questions are now being asked as to whether it is really necessary for so many births in the mid-eighties to be by the abdominal route. As the caesarean section rate is determined mainly by difficulties that arise for the first time during the course of labour in hitherto normal women, a separate chapter is devoted to this association. And because particular emphasis is placed on a correct initial diagnosis as the most important single item in management of labour, an additional chapter is addressed to the exact meaning of the term 'dilatation of cervix', a process which is of enormous practical importance in the working environment. The definitive study of intrapartum electronic fetal monitoring recently conducted in this hospital by Dr Dermot MacDonald and his colleagues is referred to under Care of Fetus. The background information, which provides an opportunity for the reader to relate aspirations expressed in the text to actual results achieved in practice, is updated to include 1984: we are indebted to Dr MacDonald and to Dr John Stronge for permission to incorporate the figures for 1977–83 and 1984, respectively. A special word of appreciation is due to Miss Evelyn Keohane for her expertise in preparing the copy.

Kieran O'Driscoll   *Declan Meagher*

Preface to the First Edition

The authors are indebted to very many persons, too numerous to mention, for advice over the years. First, it must be said that a project of this nature could not even have been contemplated without the whole-hearted co-operation of the Nursing sisters in the delivery unit, whose high standards of professional achievement were matched by a flexible attitude to new ideas to a degree that made everything possible. Likewise, our junior medical colleagues, who occupied the position of Assistant Master and whose names have appeared as co-authors of several publications in the medical press: they shared the responsibility for the welfare of every woman and delivered child and made many contributions to the underlying philosophy. And our medical colleagues farther afield, of whom a few only are mentioned here by name, because they made specific recommendations which we have incorporated as standard practice in the management of labour: Dr E. A. Friedman for the graphic representation of cervical dilatation, Dr R. H. Philpott for the introduction of an action-line, and Dr C. H. Hendricks for the suggestion that the duration of labour be measured from the time of admission to a delivery unit. We also wish to achnowledge our debt to the staff of the Physiotherapy Department and to the staff of the Medical Records Department for valuable assistance through the years. Finally, we are grateful to Dr Dermot MacDonald, presently Master of the National Maternity Hospital, for his encouragement in this undertaking.

Kieran O'Driscoll
Master
National Maternity Hospital
1963–1969

Declan Meagher
Master
National Maternity Hospital
1970–1976

DEDICATED TO THE NURSING STAFF

IN THE DELIVERY UNIT OF THE

NATIONAL MATERNITY HOSPITAL

IN RECOGNITION OF THEIR

UNFAILING CO-OPERATION AT ALL TIMES

Introduction

The purpose of this manual is to present the principles, the practice and the results of Active Management of Labour as it has evolved at the National Maternity Hospital, Dublin over a period of 22 years. The contents represent the fruits of the personal experience of the authors, who as consecutive Masters, each for seven years, were directly responsible for 86 386 births and who for the next eight years were closely involved with an additional 66 619 births: a total of 153 005 births overall. The text encompasses a comprehensive approach to the problem of labour as put into effect several times every day in the largest obstetric unit in the British Isles. This is not an academic exercise nor a review of the literature. The contents are addressed primarily to obstetricians and midwives, as the persons most closely involved with the provision of high standards of care—especially for mothers—in labour, but are hardly less relevant to anaesthetists and physiotherapists, and indeed others who strive towards this end. Also, as no expert knowledge is needed to comprehend the universal significance of the principles enunciated, the text is suitable for medical students and pupil midwives in contact with the birth process for the first time. Although the principles of Active Management of Labour remain valid in all circumstances, the practice should be considered only in the context of a suitable hospital environment, never in the home.

BACKGROUND

Although childbirth has long ceased to present a serious physical challenge to healthy women in Western society, the emotional impact of labour remains a matter of universal concern. In orthodox medical circles recognition has come slowly that labour, especially first labour, is the most disturbing emotional event in the lifetime of one-half of mankind. Failure to place nearly enough emphasis on this aspect of the subject is often attributed to the fact that obstetricians are mostly men, although midwives, as women, have shown no greater insight. Rather the correct explanation seems to be that for far too long there has been a tacit acceptance of the conservative, or passive, attitude to labour, where nothing could be done to resolve an admittedly unpleasant situation without the introduction of serious extraneous hazards with possible adverse effects on both mother and child. According to this viewpoint, which still gains wide credence, there is no safe alternative to the well-tried doctrine of watchful expectancy. But only to a point: the point of full dilatation. The doctrine of watchful expectancy covers the tedious hours of the first stage of labour until the cervix reaches full dilatation. At this point the outlook tends to change dramatically, so that almost any procedure aimed at vaginal delivery becomes acceptable. This sudden change from an extremely conservative approach to the first stage to an equally radical approach to the second stage epitomizes Passive Management of Labour, which the authors have long since abandoned. As might be expected from the foregoing, Passive Management of Labour is marked also by the emphasis placed on drugs to relieve pain during the extended first stage and on the acquisition of manual skills to procure vaginal delivery once the cervix is no longer an issue.

As the problem of maternal mortality recedes further into history, medical attention has been transferred to the child. Perinatal mortality and to an increasing degree perinatal morbidity have become the touchstones of modern obstetrics. One result of this change is that labour nowadays is made even more arduous for mothers by the introduction of invasive procedures undertaken in the name of the child, often with scant evidence as to their real value. Somehow the idea seems to have gained ground that a conflict of interest necessarily exists between mother and child during labour and that mothers can be subjected to almost any form of indignity or discomfort provided this is well-intentioned and undertaken on behalf of the child. We certainly do not subscribe to this proposition; rather, our experience suggests that what is good for mothers is also good for children, especially where short duration of labour and delivery without trauma are concerned. A main aim of this manual is to redress the rapidly growing imbalance in the birth process to favour the mother without detriment to her child.

As long ago as 1963 there began a concerted effort to improve the quality of care extended to all women in labour in this hospital. It so happens that this hospital was in an exceptionally favourable position to embark on such a project, for two main reasons: first, it was the largest maternity unit in the British Isles, and second, one obstetrician was ultimately responsible for the care of all mothers and their children. These advantages afforded a unique opportunity to establish a uniform pattern of care in a large number of cases. Two additional features are worthy of note: dead babies were invariably submitted to expert post-mortem examination, and live babies with evidence of cerebral dysfunction were placed on permanent record. Finally, there was an efficient system of medical records, which was reflected in the timely publication of an Annual Clinical Report with extensive circulation. Today, a continuous internal audit ensures that every important aspect of obstetric practice is kept under constant review, so that labour is not considered as a subject in isolation from all other aspects of childbirth, as for example caesarean section, the incidence of which remains below 5%.

Meanwhile, a growing tendency to resolve the problems of the first stage of labour by surgical intervention has resulted in an alarming increase in the number of caesarean sections performed in other centres. Caesarean section rates are currently the most realistic objective measure of the standard of obstetric care afforded to mothers, replacing maternal mortality rates, which are outmoded for this purpose in developed countries. By this criterion the standard of care afforded to mothers has declined markedly in recent years. Perinatal mortality rates must continue to serve the same purpose in infants until such time as perinatal morbidity rates are sufficiently clearly defined.

PROCEDURE

Before any worthwhile improvement in the conduct of labour could even be contemplated, it soon became clear that the person ultimately responsible must return to the delivery unit to assume direct responsibility, not just in theory but also in practice, for the welfare of all. Whereas previously the consultant obstetrician had been involved only with a small number of abnormal cases, such as those with eclampsia, breech presentation or diabetes, who happened to be in labour, he now had to become involved with the much larger number of perfectly normal women who had hitherto been overlooked at consultant level because they suffered from no organic disease. Furthermore, it was clear that this commitment must begin at admission and continue until delivery. The consultant, rather than remain off-stage, waiting for a summons to perform an emergency operation in a belated attempt to retrieve a situation that could have been anticipated at a much earlier stage, now had to seek to prevent such emergencies arising in women who were normal when they first entered hospital in labour. Ironically, it is in normal women that most of the problems of labour arise.

The position of the sister in charge of the delivery unit was a matter of no less importance. Although closely involved at all stages of labour, she remained largely powerless to influence the course of events. Apart from analgesic drugs, she lacked clear guidance on how to proceed when storm clouds began to gather. Yet, in spite of this, she was constantly exposed to the possibility of unfair criticism from either side. These genuine grievances contributed to a generally low state of morale among nursing staff, and this is one of the root causes of the relatively poor standards of overall care in many delivery units. One of the most important issues raised in this book is the urgent need to define the professional relationships that should exist between doctors and midwives at different levels of experience. Only when this issue is resolved will it be possible to develop a team spirit, which is an essential feature of good management. The adoption of good resolutions to improve the quality of care offered to all women in labour is worthless without the unqualified co-operation of nursing staff because it is the nursing staff who must convert resolutions into practice.

The delivery unit was designated an intensive care area, within which every woman and unborn child was to be reviewed by a competent doctor, in the company of the sister in charge, at regular intervals, especially late at night and early in the morning. The official record of each individual delivered during the previous 24 hours was made the object of special scrutiny by one of the authors and a running account of the main events was maintained on a daily basis. In this way the consultant obstetrician became actively involved in the conduct of labour on a regular basis as never before; hence, the origin of the term 'Active Management of Labour'. The word 'active' refers to the nature of the involvement of the consultant obstetrician and is not intended to convey to the reader that he intervenes more often. Indeed, precisely the opposite is the case, as the unusually low figures for all forms of operative intervention clearly illustrate. The active participation in the day-to-day functions of the delivery unit of the person ultimately responsible provided a new perspective on labour management and led to a fundamental reappraisal of almost all the conventional wisdoms, many of which proved to be false. Although not apparently based on any factual evidence, these conventional wisdoms had been relayed from teacher to student, and from textbook to textbook, without any serious attempt at verification, until they have come to represent possibly the main impediment to progress in the field.

As a result of this extensive personal and carefully documented experience, management of labour is now based squarely on the proposition that efficient uterine action is the key to normality. A strictly pragmatic approach has shown beyond question that efficient uterine action can be provided with a very high degree of safety, subject to a small number of rules, which can be precisely stated. As a consequence of these new-found certainties, a dynamic approach based on efficient uterine action has replaced the old static approach based largely on pelvic architecture. What may well be described as the 'domino effect of efficient uterine action' has left no aspect of labour untouched and in particular has brought about a situation in which every expectant mother who attends this hospital for antenatal care is given two firm assurances, to the effect that labour will not last longer than 12 hours and that she will never be left alone, without a personal nurse by her side at all times. These two guarantees have changed the face of women's expectations of labour. Taken together they come close to the kernel of the problem of management and in practice they are entirely dependent on each other.

PRESENTATION

This manual is divided into three sections, as follows:

Section I

This section consists of a description of the aspects of labour which the authors consider to be of such fundamental importance that each must be examined in considerable detail before any genuine progress can be made. The items are listed in the Contents and special attention should be paid to them as they are topics not often discussed in standard textbooks. Not one of them can be omitted because, like the various pieces of a jigsaw puzzle, they fit snugly together to form a composite picture of which no one fragment can stand alone. The language used is simple and direct; technical and latinate terms have purposely been avoided because they frequently only serve as a cloak to obscure the true meaning.

In the opening chapters attention is directed to the absolute need to distinguish clearly between first and subsequent births and between induction of labour and acceleration of labour that has already started, and also to the fact that obstetrical abnormalities—specifically malpresentations, malformations and twins—must always be excluded before consideration can be given to management of labour as a distinct entity. Hence this manual is concerned with the prototype of a woman in labour: the primigravida with a vertex presentation and a single fetus. In subsequent chapters the basic parameters of labour are carefully defined and the rules that govern the use of oxytocin to accelerate progress when labour is slow are stated in explicit terms.

In later chapters the causes of abnormal labour are examined and in the course of this examination the conventional approach to cephalopelvic disproportion, which has so dominated attitudes towards labour in times past, is totally rejected. Several chapters are devoted to consideration of the age-old problem of maternal stress and here the emphasis is on communication as a vital ingredient of good labour management. Drugs are found to play but a minor and largely unsatisfactory role.

The closing chapters are concerned with the organization of a busy delivery unit, where medical efficiency and human compassion can exist side-by-side. Organization is regarded as a matter of pivotal importance on which all else must ultimately depend. Indeed, poor organization is identified as the rock on which good intentions most often founder.

A chapter on the induction of labour is included in the somewhat vain hope that it may serve to dispel at least some of the obfuscation that bedevils this topic, and there is also one on the relationship between effacement and dilatation of the cervix, since these expressions are in constant use but seldom defined. Finally, there is the matter of caesarean section rates, which seem sure to develop into one of the most contentious medical issues of this decade.

A few terms may benefit from being defined because of different interpretation in other centres: a primigravida or nullipara refers to a woman who has not previously given birth to a viable infant; a nurse and a midwife are synonymous as both are state registered nurses and either trained or pupil midwives; a senior resident requires a specialist qualification in obstetrics and gynaecology.

Section II

The second section consists of a series of visual case records, each selected to illustrate one important aspect of labour, with a brief explanatory note on the facing page. These visual records, or partographs, illustrate better than words can ever do the problems that arise in the course of everyday practice. Together they constitute an identikit with which it is possible to construct an endless variety of profiles of labour, to meet almost any clinical circumstance. The authors regard this as the most important section of the book because by concentrating the mind it involves the reader directly in the study of labour as a concrete rather than an abstract pursuit.

The design and content of these visual records are matters that have an immediate effect on the conduct of labour. The model used in this hospital is worthy of close attention because it is the final product of several years of gradual development in the light of personal experience gained on the floor of a busy delivery unit. Simplicity is the keynote and every detail not immediately relevant to the main issue is rigorously excluded. The graph that portrays progress dominates the picture and no provision is made for labour to last longer than 12 hours. Two colours are used to separate primigravidae from multigravidae. This is a basic requirement. The point is emphasized again and again in the course of the text. A loose-leaf arrangement facilitates retention of all visual records of labour in two clip-in folders, one for primigravidae and the other for multigravidae. These remain in the delivery unit, where they are always available for inspection and discussion. This simple device allows a continuous audit of all recorded items, which in turn provides a very effective method of central control of the service.

The educational potential of these case records is enormous. They have made a unique contribution to the general understanding of labour and have proved to be an invaluable aid in the education of both doctors and nurses, and indeed mothers also—mothers perhaps most of all where they are used as the focus of antenatal preparation for labour. In addition, they provide fertile ground for clinical research, and for postgraduate seminars, which can be conducted like exercises in map-reading where abstract names become real places as soon as they are located in relation to the surrounding terrain. A serious student can quickly compile a personal series of case records to illustrate the whole gamut of labour and in the process construct for himself a storehouse of practical information. Success in this direction is determined by the ability of visual records to speak for themselves and thus reflect a live and durable portrait of one woman and her child in labour.

Section III

Section III consists of a summary of the clinical material that passed through the National Maternity Hospital during the years when Active Management of Labour became standard practice. This information provides the factual background to the text. As events in labour seldom happen in isolation, action taken in one direction is likely to have repercussions in another. Thus, to restrict the duration of labour to 12 hours would serve no useful purpose were this to be achieved at the expense of a significant increase in the incidence of caesarean section in the case of the mother, or mortality and morbidity in the case of the child. The facts will enable readers to see for themselves that statements made in the text are not based on theoretical considerations. They also enable comparisons to be made with results from other centres. Best of all, the figures demonstrate the balance that has been achieved between one outcome of labour and another. Information of this scope is too often missing from publications that are confined to one narrow aspect of labour: epidural anaesthesia is one of many examples. This form of selective reporting can conceal a serious underlying distortion in the overall picture.

The authors see no good reason why the results presented here should not be reproduced in other centres. This does not mean that comparable results can be achieved overnight; many delivery units are so disorganized that there is no possibility of them providing an efficient service as they stand. Dublin women are not different, only better educated in the sense that they understand the simple logic of the procedure described in these pages because it has been lucidly explained to them beforehand. This has nothing whatever to do with regimentation, rather it is a matter of common sense.

Publications on the subject of labour that emanated from the hospital during the same period are listed on p. 200. These correspond broadly with the chapter headings and are referred to in the text.

Finally, the authors recommend that the pages of this book be read through consecutively from beginning to end.

SECTION I

1

Primigravidae v. Multigravidae

There are fundamental differences between a first and all subsequent births. These differences are so great that they warrant the statement that primigravidae and multigravidae behave as different biological species. The actual nature of the differences between primigravidae and multigravidae must be appreciated before management of labour can be established on any kind of rational basis[2]*.

To ensure that the fundamental difference between a first and a subsequent birth are kept constantly in mind in this hospital the same labour record is printed on two colours, yellow for primigravidae and blue for multigravidae. The first item of information that confronts even the most casual observer is whether a woman in labour has or has not had a previous birth. This remarkably simple device has had a major impact on labour management (Graphs 1 and 30).

A Unique Experience

The modern management of labour as it relates to the welfare of mothers is concerned primarily with emotional rather than physical stress. Labour represents a physical challenge to very few women in contemporary practice and these individuals are generally identified beforehand because they suffer from specific diseases. The birth of a first child, however, is almost surely the most profound emotional experience, for good or ill, in a lifetime. The first experience is of paramount importance because it determines the attitude to all subsequent births.

A woman who has had a happy first experience is unlikely to suffer much apprehension about a later birth, whereas a woman who has had an unhappy first experience is likely to be terrified at the prospect of a repeat performance. These fears can have serious consequences outside the narrow confines of obstetrics. They can haunt a woman for the rest of her life and affect her attitude to her husband and possibly her child. The residual effect of an unhappy first experience is typically revealed in a second pregnancy by an urgent request for an epidural anaesthetic as an opening gambit at the initial antenatal visit, in the expectation that the ordeal is likely to be repeated. Prompt accession to this request reinforces the fear for which there is absolutely no foundation in clinical practice. A first labour is unique and the sequence of events that takes place on that occasion has no relevance to later births. The lesson is simple: provide a high level of care and attention

---

*The superior numerals throughout the text refer to the numbered publications listed on p. 200.

11

first time round and a woman will require little assistance on the next occasion. Conversely, the damage inflicted by a low level of care and attention first time round is usually irreversible.

Prolonged Labour

The most distinctive feature of first labour is its duration. A first labour is longer because inefficient uterine action is common and because the genital tract has not been stretched before. This applies equally to the cervix in the first stage and to the vagina in the second stage. Slow progress in a primigravida should always be regarded as an expression of inefficient uterine action. The possibility of cephalopelvic disproportion should not be entertained until efficient uterine action has been assured.

The duration of subsequent labour is comparatively short because inefficient uterine action is rare in multigravidae and because the genital tract has been stretched on a previous occasion. Slow progress in labour in a parous woman should never be assumed to be an expression of inefficient uterine action but rather an expression of obstruction caused by a fetal complication such as malpresentation or malformation. This can very easily lead to rupture of the uterus, especially where oxytocin has been used to expedite delivery.

Cephalopelvic Disproportion

Another distinctive feature of first labour is cephalopelvic disproportion. The possibility of this arises simply because the functional capacity of the pelvis is not yet known. The term 'cephalopelvic disproportion' should be restricted to primigravidae to avoid confusion with obstructed labour in multigravidae, in whom the functional capacity of the pelvis is already proven. Obstructed labour, in a multigravida, is a different clinical entity altogether and one that is fraught with far more serious consequences for both mother and child. Cephalopelvic disproportion is erroneously linked, at least in the subconscious minds of obstetricians, with fear of serious injury to mother and child. This mistaken association of ideas has impeded the management of labour for many years.

Rupture of the Uterus

Another distinctive feature of first labour is immunity to rupture. Rupture of the uterus is such an exceptional event in primigravidae that for practical purposes it can be assumed not to occur. The sole exception is manipulation. Primigravidae do not cause serious injury to themselves. Serious injury to a primigravida, of which rupture of the uterus is the ultimate expression, is caused by instruments. This is one of the most important clinical observations in the whole field of obstetrics. It has led us to a complete reappraisal of the general assumption that oxytocin may cause rupture of the uterus in the presence of cephalopelvic disproportion. There is now ample evidence that this assumption, which has dominated the conduct of labour for so long, has no foundation. There can be no doubt whatever that the mistake arose from a failure to draw a clear distinction between primigravidae and multigravidae in labour. The fear that oxytocin may cause rupture of the uterus is only too well founded in multigravidae. Whereas primigravidae are rupture-proof, multigravidae are rupture-prone. The inherent tendency of the multigravid uterus to rupture is a factor that must be taken into account whenever the subject of epidural anaesthesia is under consideration.

Traumatic Intracranial Haemorrhage

Yet another distinctive feature of first labour is the likelihood of serious injury to the child. Rupture of tentorium cerebelli with consequent subdural haemorrhage is the classic example of this. The lesion corresponds with rupture of the uterus in the mother. Rupture of the tentorium occurs during the second stage of labour, and breech presentation apart it is associated almost invariably with forceps delivery. Serious injury to the child occurs much more often in primigravidae, not because of cephalopelvic disproportion but because of the comparatively high incidence of forceps delivery. The subject of epidural anaesthesia is also relevant here.

Extensive experience with oxytocin to ensure efficient uterine action, in primigravidae, has shown that the risk of serious injury to both mother and child has been reduced because the need for forceps delivery has fallen. The risk of injury declines when babies are born by propulsion rather than traction. Trauma is discussed as a separate item in Chapter 14 (see Tables 4 and 5).

Summary

No overall plan of management for labour can hope to succeed unless it starts from the premise that primigravidae and multigravidae are radically different in almost every material respect. Inefficient uterine action is by far the most common complication of childbirth and is why long and difficult labour occurs much more often in primigravidae. The parous uterus, on the other hand, is a highly efficient organ and whenever labour proves troublesome in a multigravida the explanation should always be sought in obstruction.

One of the fundamental truths in clinical obstetrics is that the primigravid uterus is virtually immune to rupture whether or not oxytocin is used. The primigravida and her child are much more likely to have trauma inflicted on them by manipulation because of the greater need for instrumental delivery.

Finally, probably the most pervasive error in the whole of obstetrics is the practice of extrapolating from a first to a second labour. This results in treating last year's disease. There is absolutely no connection.

2

Induction v. Acceleration

Just as there are fundamental differences between first and subsequent labour, so there are fundamental differences between induction and acceleration. There exists quite a remarkable degree of confusion between these two procedures, despite the fact that appreciation of the essential differences is a prerequisite to a rational approach to management of labour. Failure to make a sufficiently sharp distinction between an attempt to interrupt the course of pregnancy, on the one hand, and to augment the course of labour as a physiological process that has already begun, on the other hand, has misled doctors, nurses and patients into the vague assumption that induction and acceleration are mere extensions of the same procedure, merging imperceptibly one into the other. This confusion stems mainly from the fact that the membranes are ruptured artificially and oxytocin is infused in both instances. The logic of this position is comparable to a conclusion that no distinction need be drawn between diseases so totally dissimilar as amoebic dysentery and trichomonal vaginitis because the therapeutic agent, metronidazole, is the same.

Duration of Stress

Induction has the direct opposite effect to acceleration because it extends the period of stress to which a woman is exposed by the time that elapses before labour begins. And this of course may not happen. As the main purpose of acceleration is to limit the period of stress to which a woman is exposed, there is an obvious need to examine very closely indeed all aspects of a procedure that has precisely the opposite effect.

Diagnosis of Labour

The diagnosis of labour is often hopelessly obscured by induction. The explanation for this is that artificial rupture of membranes is performed as part of the procedure, after which painful uterine contractions are stimulated with oxytocin. Even in normal circumstances painful uterine contractions are not reliable evidence of labour, but when they occur in response to oxytocin they should be regarded with even greater suspicion. The pains caused by oxytocin are likely to cease should the oxytocin be withdrawn. Hence it is a mistake to base a diagnosis of labour on evidence of painful uterine contractions, together with a 'show' or ruptured membranes as· in spontaneous labour. The diagnosis of labour in a case of induction rests on dilatation of the cervix alone. The result is that it is impossible to state when, if indeed ever, induction ends and labour begins. The fundamental importance of a correct initial diagnosis in management of labour is discussed at length in Chapter 5, where it is stated that diagnosis is the single most important item in management, and furthermore that whenever the diagnosis is wrong everything that follows is likely to compound the error. Nowhere is this more obvious than in cases of induction.

Operative Intervention

There is also a sharp increase in the rate of operative intervention in cases of induction. Caesarean sections performed after induction more often than not are attributed to complications of labour, such as inefficient uterine action, cephalopelvic disproportion or occipitoposterior position, when the reality is that labour has not even started. The explanation is to be found in the mistaken belief that labour begins when a woman on oxytocin complains of painful uterine contractions. Alternatively, caesarean sections performed after induction are attributed to the indications for which the inductions were performed, such as pre-eclampsia or prolonged pregnancy, although these indications seldom bear close scrutiny and would rarely justify caesarean section. There is a natural reluctance to acknowledge the fact that caesarean section is needed to retrieve a situation that stems from medical intervention, especially when the indication for this intervention lacks substance.

Favourable comparisons are sometimes made between the caesarean section rates in cases in which labour is induced and in cases in which labour is not induced. These are false because they do not compare like with like. All elective caesarean sections are included in the cases not induced and the decision to induce labour is made in the expectation of vaginal delivery. This means that the caesarean section rate in induced cases should be considerably lower than that in cases not induced and that any excess should be attributed to the procedure itself and separately recorded under the title of failed induction. The forceps rate is also higher, while, in addition, forceps are more often applied soon after full dilatation has been achieved because of the extended period of stress to which the woman has been exposed. For this reason rotation is more likely to be required. Acceleration of labour, on the other hand, reduces the rate of operative delivery because labours being shorter, mothers are more likely to deliver themselves.

Analgesia

There is a sharp increase in demand for pain relief in cases of induction. This is reflected in the dosage of drugs used and in the number of epidurals given. The increase in demand for analgesia is a measure of the increase in intensity and duration of stress caused. A surfeit of drugs raises additional problems, which are discussed in later chapters. Acceleration of labour, on the other hand, reduces the demand for analgesia because labour has already begun before anything is needed and then steps are taken to ensure that delivery occurs within a reasonable period of time.

Effects on Others

A high rate of induction subjects not only those who are directly involved to a period of stress that is prolonged artificially, its adverse effects extend to all women in labour. A high rate of induction has an important indirect bearing on other women because the resources of a delivery unit—especially the human resources—are dissipated in the care of women who are not them-selves in labour. This dilution of personal attention, which is a cornerstone of good management, affects everyone in labour and is at complete variance with the concept of intensive care. It is a strange paradox of contemporary practice that women who are not in labour should receive more attention and for a longer time than women who are in labour.

Time and Place

To ensure that the distinction between induction and acceleration is main-tained, induction is undertaken as an elective procedure at a fixed time each day in this hospital. Emergency inductions are not permitted. Moreover, the artificial rupture of membranes, to induce labour, is performed in another place and the patient returns to an antenatal ward to await labour. A firm diagnosis of labour is mandatory before amniotomy can be performed or oxytocin infused in the delivery unit. Hence time and place are used to reinforce the message. This ensures that clear decisions are made, especially in respect of the diagnosis of labour, before any intervention is allowed. The rationale is comparable to the use of different coloured charts to separate primigravidae from multigravidae, as described in the previous chapter. The induction and acceleration of labour are discussed as separate items in Chapters 8 and 24.

Summary

Induction has several adverse effects on the conduct of labour. Emotional and physical stress are both increased. The diagnosis of labour is confused. The operative intervention rate is increased. There is greater demand for analgesia. The quality of care offered to all mothers is diluted. As this is a formidable list, cases of induction should always be reported separately so that full implications of this form of intervention can be seen.

3

Malpresentations, Malformations, Twins

The third fundamental distinction that must be drawn before labour can be discussed in a rational manner is that between the management of labour and the treatment of obstetric abnormalities. This manual on the management of labour is confined to cases in which there is a single fetus, a vertex presentation and a normal head. Obstetric abnormalities, particularly those that involve the fetus directly, are specifically excluded from consideration because they may cause obstruction during labour and place the fetus and sometimes the mother at risk. Treatment of obstetric abnormalities including malpresentations, malformations and twins is discussed at length in the standard textbooks, where little attention is paid to management of labour as a separate entity. These topics are as much outside the scope of the present book as are obstetric abnormalities that involve the mother directly, such as eclampsia or postpartum haemorrhage.

A brief outline of the general approach to the treatment of malpresentations, malformations and twins in this hospital is given in this chapter. All subsequent chapters are written on the assumption that definitive steps have been taken to exclude these conditions beforehand. Some 95% of admissions are still included.

Breech and Face Presentations

The hazards of breech delivery are confined to the child. Virtually the only danger to the mother is through medical intervention. The approach to the treatment of breech presentation in labour is entirely pragmatic. Vaginal delivery is preferred whenever this can be accomplished without medical intervention. Caesarean section is the only form of treatment allowed, whether the need should arise during the first or second stage of labour. Oxytocin is never used to accelerate progress in breech presentation. X-ray pelvimetry is not practised, since the size and shape of the pelvis are not factors that are taken into account in deciding the mode of delivery.

The approach to face presentation is along similar lines. Vaginal delivery is preferred whenever this can be accomplished without medical intervention. Caesarean section is the only form of treatment allowed. Oxytocin is never used to accelerate progress in face presentation.

Brow and Shoulder Presentations

Brow presentation and shoulder presentation—the latter a rare occurrence in primigravidae—are treated always by caesarean section. These are two of the notable causes of obstructed labour that can so easily lead to rupture of the uterus in multigravidae. Hence, brow and shoulder presentation differ from breech and face presentation in that they place the life of the mother at risk. Treatment of malpresentations by manipulation is not practised in this hospital. Naturally oxytocin is not used.

Hydrocephalus

The only malformation likely to cause obstruction is hydrocephalus. This is the third notable cause of obstructed labour that leads to rupture of the uterus in multigravidae. The condition is treated by simple aspiration through a spinal needle sometimes through the mother's abdomen, after which labour is allowed to proceed. Oxytocin of course is not used.

Twins

Twins are regarded as an obstetric abnormality mainly because the second twin is exposed to special hazards during the course of labour. The second twin may suffer the effects of hypoxia because, not being so readily accessible, he/she cannot be properly supervised. Not infrequently, he/she may be a victim of chronic placental insufficiency, with retarded growth, resorption of liquor and passage of meconium, none of which is suspected until the membranes rupture after the first twin is born, when it may be too late to take effective action. Furthermore, the second twin may become misplaced, typically as a shoulder presentation, after the first twin is born. Slow labour in twins is treated always by caesarean section. Oxytocin is never used.

Obstruction

Notwithstanding the fact that detection of malpresentations, malformations and twins is an integral part of antenatal care and that independent assessment at the point of admission is mandatory, the final responsibility rests squarely on the person who makes the decision to use oxytocin to accelerate slow labour to ensure that these complications have been excluded in each individual case. The person who prescribes oxytocin for a woman in labour should be required to place on record that the vertex presents, that the head is normal and that there is a single fetus. But in practice it is in multigravidae only that malpresentations and malformations present a serious threat to the mother, because it is in multigravidae that obstruction may lead to rupture of the uterus whether or not oxytocin is used. The reason why oxytocin should be used with extreme caution, if ever, in multigravidae is that the parous uterus is highly vulnerable in this regard. This is certainly not true in primigravidae. Inadvertently over the years oxytocin has been given to primigravidae with obstructed labour caused by malpresentations and malformations without untoward effect. This is of course a culpable error.

The three classical causes of abnormal labour—inefficient uterine action, occipitoposterior position and cephalopelvic disproportion—are not regarded as obstetric abnormalities. They are aberrations which arise in normal cases after admission to hospital in labour. This is a point of great practical importance because there are many who practise obstetrics in the belief that cephalopelvic disproportion is an obstetric abnormality that can be detected beforehand. This mistaken belief results in elective caesarian sections which are quite unnecessary and which, moreover, are wrongly reported as examples of cephalopelvic disproportion.

Summary

Every discussion on the subject of labour should be confined strictly to cases in which the vertex presents, the head is normal and there is a single fetus. The subject should not be confused by the introduction of obstetric abnormalities, particularly those that involve the fetus as a cause of obstruction. This is a common mistake. There is a serious obligation on the part of the person responsible to ensure that malpresentations, malformations and twins have been excluded before oxytocin is authorized. Obstructed labour should be recognized as a clinical entity completely different from cephalopelvic disproportion. This has particular relevance to multigravidae, in whom obstructed labour is far the most common cause of rupture of the intact uterus in all obstetric practice.

4

Duration of Labour

It would be difficult indeed to exaggerate the beneficial effects of an accurate working definition of duration of labour on clinical practice, since failure to define what is one of the basic parameters of labour has been a major obstacle to improvements in management for many years[5].

Definition

In this hospital duration of labour is defined as the number of hours a woman spends in the delivery unit from the time of her admission until the time her baby is born. No allowance is made for time spent in labour at home. Speculation on the number of hours a woman may have been in labour before she chose to admit herself to hospital is a fruitless exercise. This is an argument that cannot be resolved satisfactorily and which in any event has no relevance to clinical practice. Incidentally, the third stage is not included in this definition of labour.

There are four reasons why duration of labour is so defined:

1. The time of admission is decided by the woman herself.
2. Professional responsibility begins when a woman elects to place herself under care.
3. The duration of labour can be recorded accurately for purposes of comparison.
4. Mothers themselves tend to recall the duration of labour in this manner.

Effectively, the overall duration of labour is determined by the length of the first stage because the number of hours taken for the cervix to dilate represents some 90% of the entire birth process. The second stage is short by comparison and contributes little to the overall problem of prolonged labour.

This definition applies equally when a woman not in labour remains in the delivery unit for any reason. Hence, duration of labour in the case of a woman admitted for induction is also recorded as hours spent in the delivery unit because this is the measure of stress to which she is exposed. Although it is not possible to say at what point induction ends and labour begins, the procedure exposes the woman to the same pressures as if she were in labour all of that time. The definition applies even should induction fail and resort be made to caesarean section. Similarly, when a woman is retained in the delivery unit in error because of a wrong diagnosis of labour, duration is still recorded from the time of admission. This means that duration of labour is entered for some women who are recognized in retrospect as not having been in labour at all and it shows the extent to which duration is synonymous with time spent in the delivery unit of the hospital.

Advantages of Short Labour

The mean duration of first labour—without any form of medical intervention—is somewhat less than six hours in this hospital. Women in general tolerate the stress of labour of this duration very well, and provided that they have a reasonable understanding of what to expect and are not left alone at any time, they require little in the way of analgesia and usually succeed in delivering themselves.

To the mother

The impact of labour must be evaluated as much in emotional as in physical terms. Both are more closely related to the number of hours spent in a delivery unit than to any other measurable factor. Some women are already unduly perturbed at the point of admission, while others remain apparently unmoved after many hours; but most fall somewhere between these two extremes. The morale of the average woman begins to deteriorate perceptibly after six hours. After 12 hours the deterioration accelerates rapidly—almost in geometric rather than arithmetic progression as hitherto—until eventually a stage is reached at which an adult is reduced to pleading for deliverance from passers-by unless she is rendered semiconscious with drugs or lulled into a false sense of security with epidural anaesthesia. It cannot be over-emphasized that the profound emotional disturbance caused by prolonged labour may endure for a lifetime. Consequently, no woman should be permitted to continue long enough in labour to need more than two standard doses of analgesia by whatever method these are administered. Exogenous influences, other than time, that have a significant bearing on the emotional equilibrium of women in labour are good antenatal education, continuous personal attention and proper use of drugs to relieve pain. These items are discussed at length in subsequent chapters.

To these enormously important, if somewhat less tangible, emotional benefits must be added the physical benefits of short labour. Nowadays no one need be permitted to continue long enough in labour to suffer from dehydration, ketosis or salt depletion. There is virtually no possibility of these disturbances arising within a time-scale of 12 hours. These considerations assume even greater relevance in warmer climes, where changes of this nature occur so much more rapidly. There are also the very considerable advantages of a lesser need for surgical intervention, notably caesarean section during the first stage and rotational forceps during the second stage, simply because fit mothers are much better able to deliver themselves. Lastly there is a greatly reduced demand for analgesic drugs which means that mothers retain ultimate control.

To the child

Duration of labour is equally important for the child. A fetus is exposed to the risk of hypoxia mainly in the first stage and of trauma mainly in the second stage. There is an especially close correlation between trauma and duration because long labours frequently end in difficult forceps extractions. Previously, the medical approach to prolonged labour was based on full dilatation of the cervix as the natural line of demarcation between abdominal and vaginal delivery. The aim was to sustain the mother, and through her hopefully also the baby, until full dilatation was reached. Full dilatation became an end in itself and when this was achieved the common ordeal was brought to a speedy and often forcible conclusion. This meant that forceps were applied before the head could descend to the level at which rotation into the anterior position normally occurs. Not infrequently serious trauma was inflicted in the process. The circle of confusion was complete when the difficult extraction and consequent trauma were interpreted as evidence that prolonged labour is a common expression of cephalopelvic disproportion. Emphatically, this is *not* so.

To the staff

Duration of labour is a matter that affects professional staff greatly too. A sense of impotence in the face of widespread physical suffering and even moral degradation frequently colours the attitude of midwives and doctors from their early student days. Those who subsequently specialize react in different ways: obstetricians tend to avoid the delivery unit as much as possible, while midwives left to themselves tend to resort to excessive use of analgesia and epidural anaesthesia. Control of duration of labour is almost as important for midwives as it is for mothers and babies.

To the administrators

Duration of labour is a matter of great importance to administrators too, because the delivery unit represents the bottleneck in a maternity service through which all the consumers must pass. The result is that it is not possible to plan maternity hospital accommodation or to allocate nursing staff, in particular, on a rational basis unless the number of patient-hours to be serviced can be calculated in advance. This is a prime example of the application of cost-efficiency in contemporary medical practice, where good medicine and sound economics complement each other. Nowhere is this seen to better advantage than in a modern efficient intensive-care delivery unit.

Conclusion

Prolonged labour in this hospital was defined as 36 hours in 1963, reduced to 24 hours in 1968 and finally to 12 hours in 1972. A formal decision to restrict the duration of labour to 12 hours was introduced on 1 January 1972. Since then no provision has been made on the official record for labour to last a longer time. The result is a declared policy, of which all expectant mothers are made fully aware, not to expose anyone to the stress of labour for more than 12 hours. Meanwhile, well in excess of 100 000 babies have been born. Every mother not close to an easy vaginal delivery after 12 hours is submitted to caesarean section. Contrary to expectations this practice has not led to an increase in the use of caesarean section, which remains at the comparatively low level of 5% of all births. What may have appeared lost on the swings has been more than recovered on the roundabouts. The deeper implications of the consistently low incidence of caesarean section as compared with the startling increase in most other centres over the same period are considered in Chapter 27.

Summary

Duration is the kernel of the problem of management of labour. More than any other measurable factor, duration determines the impact on mothers in particular, but also on babies, and on all those who care for both of them. Duration of labour should be equated with hours spent in a delivery unit. The ability to restrict the duration of labour without extending the use of caesarian section represents a major advance in obstetric practice. This is also evident in the total abolition of dehydration, ketosis and salt depletion, and a dramatic reduction in demand for analgesia. There is a parallel decline in the need for instrumental delivery, especially rotational forceps, because given labour of short duration, women are much better able to cope and eventually to deliver themselves. Finally, duration is essentially a problem of first labour. (See Figure 1.)

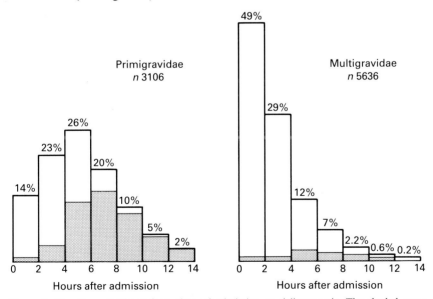

Figure 1. Duration of labour from time of admission to delivery unit. The shaded areas represent the proportion of patients receiving oxytocin: multigravidae include first vaginal deliveries after previous caesarean section[15].

5

Diagnosis of Labour

The most important single item in the management of labour is diagnosis. When the initial diagnosis is wrong, all subsequent management is likely to be wrong also. The unfortunate consequences of this are to be seen almost daily in our delivery units, although they are seldom recognized for what they are. In medical circles there is an almost universal failure to appreciate that the diagnosis of labour presents a genuine problem. This has led to an altogether anomalous situation, in which the fundamental decision on which all subsequent management is based is surrendered to the patients. Uniquely, an expectant mother admits herself to a maternity hospital, with the result that she tends to dictate her own treatment. This procedure, which leaves the initiative in the hands of the patients, has no parallel in other branches of medicine.[8]

Doctors and nurses are noticeably vague whenever questions are asked about the diagnosis of labour. Hence it should come as no surprise that mothers, especially primigravidae with no previous experience, should sometimes be mistaken and admit themselves to hospital in error. Perhaps the most surprising feature of all is not that mothers are sometimes wrong but that they are usually right.

There are very few maternity centres indeed where any serious attention is paid to the diagnosis of labour. The general assumption is that no such problem exists, because women are naturally equipped with an unerring instinct that enables them to make a correct decision in these matters. The subject is not discussed in textbooks and is evaded in medical publications where only cases said to be established in labour, because the cervix is well dilated, are included in reports. The alternative practice is to resort to the very simple device of making a retrospective decision that a woman was in labour because her baby has been born. In everyday clinical practice, however, decisions must be prospective; medicine in real life does not include the luxury of wisdom after the event. An essential difference between the theory and the practice of medicine is that the doctor—or more likely the nurse—does not enjoy the benefit of hindsight when an agitated woman presents herself at a delivery unit late at night because she thinks she is in labour. A firm decision is needed in these circumstances. Equivocal terms such as false labour, latent labour and labour that is not established serve only as strategems to relieve the doctor—or nurse—of the onus of having to make this decision. Such terms have no real meaning, but the effect is to pass the responsibility for the diagnosis of labour back to the patient, where it certainly does not belong. Most errors in management

24

of labour result from decisions avoided rather than from decisions wrongly made. This dictum applies with particular force to the initial diagnosis.

The First Step

The first step in the management of labour is to confirm or deny the presumptive diagnosis that has been made by the patient prior to admission. There are strict instructions to this effect in this hospital. These must be put into practice not later than one hour after admission. The sister in charge of the delivery unit is nominated as the person directly responsible. The official labour chart is designed in such a manner as to ensure that the evidence on which her decision is based is placed on permanent record. The terms are both simple and explicit. This evidence is placed in a prominent position. Thus a prospective diagnosis of labour is made in every case admitted and the evidence on which this was based remains always available, even when the sister in question has gone off duty (see Graph 3).

Incidentally, no treatment of any sort is permitted until a firm diagnosis of labour has been made because treatment of any kind commits a woman to delivery whether or not she is in labour. Naturally, whenever a woman's presumptive diagnosis of labour is not accepted, she deserves an adequate explanation, which should be couched in simple language that she can easily comprehend. The explanation given in this hospital is a mere paraphrase of what is written here and it is almost universally well received. The woman is then transferred to an antenatal ward, where she is retained until the next day. A woman who is adjudged not in labour is not retained in the delivery unit one moment longer than is necessary and never longer than one hour. But neither is she allowed home, lest the passage of time should prove her diagnosis to have been correct, which inevitably sometimes happens.

Pains

A woman's diagnosis of labour is based on the subjective element of pain. Pain is such a constant feature that without pain the question of labour simply does not arise. However, not every woman who complains of pain is necessarily in labour, although late in pregnancy some, not unnaturally, are likely to think that they are. The nature and distribution of the pain may be so uncharacteristic that it bears no resemblance to labour, in which case it can be readily discounted by the experienced observer. Alternatively, the pain may be so characteristic—intermittent and symmetrical, as well as coincident with uterine contractions—that it makes for a more difficult decision.

There is a popular misconception even in medical circles that pain that coincides with uterine contractions provides conclusive evidence of labour. This is an elementary mistake. A doctor or nurse with a hand on the abdomen to confirm that a woman winces as her uterus contracts needs to appreciate that Braxton Hicks' contractions, which are a normal feature of late pregnancy, increase in both strength and frequency as term approaches and, furthermore, that they can cause considerable discomfort when the threshold for pain is low. Pain of this nature cannot be distinguished from the pain of labour because of the common origin. The threshold for pain is reduced mainly through anxiety, which is most likely to occur late at night, especially when a woman is alone or resides at a considerable distance from the hospital. Understandably, a woman who fears that she may arrive too late tends to travel too early. These are important factors, which should be taken into account when considering a diagnosis of labour.

An air of uncertainty at the point of admission compounds the problem further because the woman quickly senses that the experts from whom she had the right to expect guidance cannot even diagnose labour. Instead of firm direction she meets with evasion and this undermines her confidence all the more. As anxiety increases, the pain gets worse. Unfortunately, the staff are wont to respond with analgesic drugs, which have the indirect effect of committing the woman to delivery. Therefore it must be made absolutely clear that painful uterine contractions alone do not warrant a medical diagnosis of labour. Painful uterine contractions must be supported by evidence of a more objective kind before a medical diagnosis of labour can be upheld.

Effacement and Dilatation

The diagnosis of labour presents no problem whatever when painful uterine contractions are combined with dilatation of the cervix because the very essence of labour is the opening of the neck of the womb. A woman who enters hospital with her cervix well dilated is not only surely in labour but can be expected to proceed rapidly and to deliver within a matter of a few hours. Moreover, the extent of dilatation of the cervix at the point of admission is a clear indication of the efficiency of uterine action and not, as often supposed, a reflection of the number of hours spent in labour at home. Reports in the medical press that are confined to cases in which labour is said to be established not only evade the fundamental question of diagnosis but likewise exclude from consideration the very cases that are likely to cause problems in management. Because these are the women who suffer from inefficient uterine action, such selective reporting has no real value in practice.

As dilatation of the cervix affords the sole conclusive evidence of labour, it is clearly essential that this term be accurately defined. Inevitably this also entails definition of the term effacement, because the two are so closely related and often confused. Chapter 26 is devoted to consideration of these important items in greater detail. Meanwhile, effacement refers to incorporation of the cervical canal into the lower uterine segment. This proceeds downwards from above, that is from the internal to external os. The process may occur late in pregnancy or be delayed until labour begins. Dilatation, on the other hand, refers only to the external os. This cannot begin to open until the entire length of the canal has been obliterated, at which stage effacement is complete. As this marks the point of transition, it is a contradiction in terms to speak of dilatation before effacement is complete.

The external os is seldom so tightly closed that it does not admit a fingertip long before labour begins. This can be a cause of confusion when a fingertip is equated with 1 cm on the notional metric scale used to express the extent of dilatation during labour. Effacement is the feature that serves to distinguish between a cervix that passively admits a fingertip and a cervix that is dilated 1 cm. A diagnosis of labour is made when a woman admits herself to this hospital with painful uterine contractions and the cervix is found, on pelvic examination, to be completely effaced. Such a woman is retained in the delivery unit and is therefore committed to delivery within 12 hours.

With regard to the diagnosis of labour, the problems are to be found among the considerable number of women who admit themselves to hospital with painful uterine contractions but in whom the cervix is not completely effaced. In these circumstances objective evidence of a different nature must be sought. A 'show' or spontaneous rupture of membranes provides the alternative. These simple signs are invaluable aids to diagnosis when the cervix is not completely effaced.

'Show'

A 'show' or blood-stained plug of mucus passed early in labour, often before effacement is complete and dilatation can begin, is easily recognized by patients and staff alike and therefore has a major role to play in the diagnosis of labour. Although not conclusive in the sense that dilatation is conclusive, a 'show' affords presumptive evidence of change in the condition of the cervix sufficient to cause the operculum to be extruded.

A firm diagnosis of labour is made in this hospital when subjective evidence of pain is supported by objective evidence of a 'show' even though the cervix may not be effaced, let alone dilated. A woman with painful uterine contractions and a 'show' is retained in the delivery unit and therefore committed to delivery in 12 hours without regard to the condition of her cervix. An exception is sometimes made in the case of a woman who is less than 37 weeks, in the somewhat vain hope that labour may be averted. A 'show' has already occurred in approximately 70% of women who admit themselves to this hospital in the belief that they are in labour.

Naturally, a 'show' without painful uterine contractions does not warrant this interpretation. A 'show' in these circumstances is recorded as unsubstantial antepartum haemorrhage and the woman is transferred to an antenatal ward. A 'show' that follows vaginal examination is regarded as an artefact about which everyone exposed is advised.

Ruptured Membranes

Spontaneous rupture of membranes is regarded as even stronger presumptive evidence of labour than a 'show'. A firm diagnosis of labour is made when a woman admits herself to this hospital with painful uterine contractions supported by spontaneous rupture of membranes. She is retained in the delivery unit and therefore committed to delivery in 12 hours without regard to the condition of her cervix. Spontaneous rupture of membranes has already occurred in approximately 30% of women who admit themselves to this hospital in the belief that they are in labour.

Similarly, spontaneous rupture of membranes alone does not warrant a diagnosis of labour. Membranes may rupture several weeks before labour begins. A woman with spontaneous rupture of membranes but without painful uterine contractions is transferred to an antenatal ward. Even when the length of gestation exceeds 42 weeks a decision to attempt to induce labour with oxytocin must be deferred at least until the next day. Induction is permitted only as an elective procedure. Emergency inductions are not allowed. This strict rule serves to maintain the sharp distinction between acceleration of labour that has already begun and initiation of labour that has not yet started. Hence the problem of diagnosis of labour must be confronted at every step. In the event of a woman with only spontaneous rupture of membranes returning to the delivery unit within a few hours, it is not concluded that the initial decision was necessarily wrong. More likely, the correct explanation is that the woman has meanwhile induced labour on herself, so to speak. Rupture of membranes, whether artificial or spontaneous, is after all an effective method of starting labour.

Vaginal examination is prohibited when there is any likelihood that a woman admitted with spontaneous rupture of membranes may not be in labour. This prohibition is to prevent the introduction of infection, which could gravely prejudice the outcome. A casual vaginal examination performed on a woman with ruptured membranes commits her to delivery whether or not she is in labour. Eventually this may require an unnecessary caesarean section. Consequently routine performance of vaginal examination at the point of admission to a delivery unit is indicative of a lack of foresight in this regard. There are additional grounds for this reservation when the duration of pregnancy is less than 37 weeks, and it seems desirable that delivery be postponed in the interest of further maturity.

A 'show' and spontaneous rupture of membranes count as independent signs of labour when the 'show' appears first, but as only one sign when the membranes rupture first because the significance of a 'show' is vitiated by prior rupture of membranes.

Errors in Diagnosis

An error in the diagnosis of labour can be made either way.

A woman's diagnosis of labour may be accepted, in which case she is retained in the delivery unit and exposed to the manifold pressures of that environment. Inevitably her morale begins to crumble and her physical condition eventually deteriorates as time passes and no progress is made. The problem is compounded by analgesic drugs or epidural block and eventually oxytocin, until a point is reached at which there is no option other than to terminate her ordeal by resort to caesarean section. The record will undoubtedly show that caesarean section was performed for maternal or fetal distress caused by prolonged labour, whereas the truth of the matter is that the initial diagnosis of labour was wrong. A state of labour never existed. The very first occasion that such a woman is seen by the obstetrician responsible may be to perform the operation. The clinical history available at this juncture is likely, at best, to be second-hand. It is usually impossible to identify the person who made the fateful decision, much less review the evidence on which that decision was based. In everyday practice these questions are seldom even asked because their significance is not appreciated.

Alternatively, a woman's diagnosis of labour may be rejected, in which case she is transferred to an antenatal ward only to return a short time later well advanced in labour. This is not a serious mistake provided that she is not sent home, and to guard against this possibility every woman who admits herself to this hospital because she thinks she is in labour is retained until the following day.

Of course it must be freely acknowledged that no matter how much careful attention is paid to the diagnosis of labour, subsequent events will sometimes prove it incorrect simply because it is not possible to make a correct decision in every case. No method is foolproof. Rather, the aim should be to reduce the number of errors to a minimum and to operate a fail-safe procedure which ensures, in so far as is possible, that when an error does occur it can be retrieved in good time, as follows.

First, the woman who is retained in the delivery unit in error. Here failure of the cervix to respond to oxytocin, which must be used eventually to rectify slow progress, should quickly raise the suspicion that a mistake has been made. Treatment should be stopped before the point of no return is reached. The position should be explained to the patient in intelligible terms and she should be transferred to an antenatal ward. This woman can be expected to return some hours later and to proceed to deliver rapidly because she is now in labour. The ability to retrieve an admittedly difficult situation like this depends partly on the sense of trust that the mother places in the staff and partly on the confidence that the staff have in themselves. Self-confidence permits mistakes to be openly acknowledged and freely discussed. These characteristics are in themselves very closely related to the standards of practice in a delivery unit. However, some mothers become so distressed by the experience that it is not possible to return to the original position, in which event caesarean section is the only solution. But the fact remains that the true state of affairs is seldom recognized. Approximately 10% of women who admit themselves to this hospital under the impression that they are in labour are mistaken. It is a matter of paramount importance that these women be identified before they find themselves on a production line from which there is generally only one escape route: caesarean section, and that after much anguish.

Second, the woman who is transferred to an antenatal ward because her diagnosis of labour is not accepted. She is not allowed home until formally discharged on the following day. This eliminates the possible embarrassment of giving birth on the way home. Incidentally, a woman who returns to the delivery unit before discharge is presumed to have been in labour at the time of first admission.

Diagnosis of Labour after Induction

Finally, a note about induction. Anyone concerned with the quality of care in labour must look very closely indeed at the practice of induction, a subject about which more is written in Chapter 24. In the present context it cannot be over-emphasized that a procedure that includes artificial rupture of membranes and infusion of oxytocin plays absolute havoc with the diagnosis of labour. Oxytocin causes painful uterine contractions whether or not a woman is in labour. This is a particular example of the serious fallacy of basing a diagnosis of labour on painful uterine contractions. In the course of an induction the significance of painful uterine contractions, a 'show' and ruptured membranes are all vitiated. Hence the diagnosis of labour in a case of induction rests solely on dilatation of the cervix. The fact that this is not generally appreciated leads to widespread confusion about when an induction ends and labour begins. Incidentally, this provides the opportunity of attributing an adverse outcome in such a case to a complication of labour rather than to a failed induction, where it properly belongs.

There is one other aspect of the problem of diagnosis of labour worthy of brief comment. This concerns claims made for treatment aimed at arresting the course of labour that has started prematurely. The credibility of many such claims rests entirely on whether or not the patients treated were in labour to begin with, that is on the accuracy of the initial diagnosis. Advocates of this form of therapy tend to start from the premise that the diagnosis of labour is such a simple matter that it can be taken for granted, which is very far from the truth. Such scant attention is paid to the problem of diagnosis of labour at term that it comes as a surprise to find the ease with which it is made prematurely in many publications advocating the benefits of tocolytic agents.[14]

Summary

Diagnosis is the single most important item in the conduct of labour. Significantly, this is the longest chapter in the book. As with every clinical problem in medicine, labour too must begin with correct diagnosis. Wrong diagnosis inevitably leads to wrong treatment. Every diagnosis must of its nature be prospective and a diagnosis of labour is, in effect, a positive decision to commit a woman to delivery. Clearly a matter of such consequence should not be left to the patient to decide.

Painful uterine contractions alone do not warrant a medical diagnosis of labour. Pains must be supported by a 'show', spontaneous rupture of membranes or dilatation of the cervix. Although dilatation of the cervix represents the only conclusive evidence of labour, in practice a 'show' or spontaneous rupture of membranes—combined with painful uterine contractions—affords sufficiently strong presumptive evidence to commit a woman to delivery. Given the importance of dilatation of the cervix, it is imperative that the term be accurately defined.

There are two common errors: first, treatment is initiated on the basis of painful uterine contractions not supported by any other evidence of labour, and second, treatment is withheld although painful uterine contractions are supported by a 'show' or spontaneous rupture of membranes because the cervix is not dilatated. There remains the possibility that subsequent events may show the initial decision to have been incorrect and this too should be kept in mind.

6

Progress: First Stage

After the diagnosis of labour has been confirmed, the next important item in management is to monitor progress at short and regular intervals, especially in the early hours. Progress during the first stage of labour is measured exclusively in terms of dilatation of the cervix because the sole function of uterine action during the first stage is to open the exit from the womb sufficiently to allow the baby's head to pass through. The rate of dilatation of the cervix is crucial because the duration of labour depends almost entirely on the duration of the first stage. This is true to such an extent that the two are almost synonymous in everyday practice. The first stage accounts for some 90% of the entire duration of labour in ordinary circumstances.

Descent of the baby's head is certainly not an appropriate measure of progress during the first stage of labour. There is no consistent relationship between dilatation of the cervix and descent of the head. Descent of the head is the measure of progress appropriate to the second stage of labour. The sole function of uterine action during the second stage is to propel the fetus along the birth canal.

Pelvic Examination

Pelvic examination is performed at the point of admission and thereafter at regular intervals of one hour for the next three hours. Subsequent examinations are performed at the discretion of the examiner but at intervals of not longer than two hours. Successive examinations are performed by the same person, in so far as possible, because there is a not inconsiderable subjective element in interpretation. Dilatation of the cervix is not capable of accurate measurement and this is one clinical situation in which too many cooks will surely spoil the broth. The sister in charge of the delivery unit is named as the person responsible for the assessment of progress, just as she is responsible for the diagnosis of labour. The subjective element in interpretation is most pronounced at times when changes of staff occur. This possibility should be kept constantly in mind because it has a practical bearing on management when a false impression of secondary arrest in progress is created.

Cervical Dilatation

The degree of dilatation of the cervix is recorded on a simple graph and plotted against hours after admission. Full dilatation is equated with 10 cm because this is the diameter of a baby's head. The maximum time allotted is 10 hours. It follows that the slowest rate of dilatation acceptable is 1 cm per hour. The whole purpose of the graph is to relate progress in labour to the passage of time in a visual manner that is readily intelligible even to a lay person. Illustrations are provided in Section II of this manual. The extent to which rate of progress dominates all other aspects of labour should be noted. Graphic records of labour are so often crammed with detail that the visual impact is completely lost, with the result that the main purpose of the exercise is obscured, if not defeated. Efforts to include every detail of every aspect of labour, whether relevant or not, are therefore counterproductive.

A clear pattern of dilatation should have emerged at the end of three hours and on this basis it should be possible to predict the hour of delivery by simple linear projection, in all but a few instances. Close attention to progress during the early hours of labour is the best insurance against trouble later. The weight of emphasis placed on the first three hours of labour stands in sharp contrast with previous practice, when no worthwhile medical decision was considered necessary until a woman had been in labour for several hours and complications had begun to arise. Those late decisions were concerned more with the rescue of mothers and babies from potentially dangerous predicaments which had developed over a protracted period of time in normal cases after admission to hospital. No thought was given to prevention.

An unsatisfactory rate of dilatation of the cervix during the early hours of labour is a clear and unequivocal expression of inefficient uterine action. This should be corrected in good time. This pattern of dilatation has no relevance whatever to cephalopelvic disproportion, a point that has given rise to a great deal of confusion in the past. Treatment of inefficient uterine action is discussed in Chapter 8 and illustrated in Graphs 19 and 20.

Communication

One of the main benefits to accrue from regular pelvic assessment at short intervals is the ability to keep the mother posted on the progress of events. Hopefully, it will have been explained to her beforehand, at antenatal classes, that the purpose of the examinations is to measure the speed at which the neck of her womb is opening, because this effectively determines the length of her labour. In that case she will be already familiar with the graph. And as time passes the result of each examination is conveyed directly to the mother by the examiner as it is being entered on the graph. Because a lay person is not well attuned to think in terms of dilatation of the cervix but merely anxious to know when her baby will be born, attention is directed to the time-scale for her benefit. The need to be convinced that steady progress is being made and to appreciate that there is a definite end in sight are matters of utmost importance to the morale of all concerned. The standard practice in this hospital is to inform every woman in labour of the expected time of her delivery as soon as a pattern of dilatation is established, which is seldom later than three hours after admission. Time of delivery is stated to within 30 minutes. A woman is told at noon that her baby is expected at four o'clock in the afternoon, give or take half an hour. This information is updated after each examination. No examination is undertaken on a woman in labour without direct reference to her before and after the event. She must know the purpose of the examination and be the first to learn of the result. The onus rests squarely on the examiner to ensure that she genuinely understands the real meaning of what is being said. Platitudes to the effect that 'all is well' or that 'progress is as good as can be expected' are not acceptable. These represent an affront to the intelligence of women generally and thus undermine mutual confidence. Similarly, technical terms are strictly avoided. These are seen to be a cloak for ignorance. An examiner who does not truly comprehend the implications of the signs elicited is in no position to explain them to someone else and therefore retreats behind medical jargon.

Rectal v. Vaginal Examination

Rectal examination is the method used to measure progress in labour in this hospital. Vaginal examination is not undertaken without special reason, such as to perform artificial rupture of membranes, exclude prolapse of the cord or when the result of rectal examination is inconclusive. Rectal examination has some advantages over vaginal examination for the purpose of routine assessment. The main advantage is that elaborate precautions against infection are not required. This is a matter of considerable practical importance in a busy unit, where several women are in labour at the same time. Rectal examination is more likely to be performed at short intervals on this account. Vaginal examination on the other hand gives rise to practical problems, with the result that progress is measured less frequently, usually at intervals of four hours. Four hours is much too long to wait to discover that labour has not progressed since a previous examination and much too long to wait to discover that treatment prescribed to accelerate slow progress after a previous examination has not been successful. Prolonged labour occurs much more frequently when pelvic examination is performed at infrequent and irregular intervals. Infrequent and irregular pelvic examinations encourage a tolerant attitude to prolonged labour. Furthermore, vaginal examination is potentially dangerous when there is a possibility of ruptured membranes in a woman who may not be in labour. A vaginal examination in these circumstances commits the woman to delivery because of risk of infection; this may result in the birth of a preterm infant or in a caesarean section that is undertaken to retrieve an iatrogenic disease. In this hospital vaginal examination is not permitted if there is any possibility of ruptured membranes, unless a firm diagnosis of labour has already been made. However, it must be conceded that rectal assessment of cervical dilatation is not always reliable even in expert hands and this may lead to a mistaken conclusion that progress is being made when this is not the case. Moreover, a recent controlled study in this hospital revealed to our surprise that women in general prefer vaginal examination. The choice of method is therefore likely to remain a matter of local custom.

Summary

The sole purpose of uterine action during the first stage of labour is to open the neck of the womb sufficiently to allow the baby to pass through. Hence dilatation of the cervix is the only measure of progress appropriate to the first stage of labour. As this proceeds uniformly it is eminently feasible to predict, a few hours after admission, the approximate time of delivery or to take prompt action against a drift into prolonged labour. Regular pelvic assessment at short intervals should be mandatory during the first three hours.

7

Progress: Second Stage

The second stage of labour begins at full dilatation. In practice this means that no part of the cervix is palpable at pelvic examination. For record purposes only, full dilatation is equated with 10 cm simply because this is the approximate width of the mature fetal skull. Progress in the second stage is measured in terms of descent, and incidentally rotation.

The contribution of the second stage to the total duration of labour is relatively small because the second stage seldom lasts longer than two hours. The second stage deserves particular attention because of the special risk of trauma. Although trauma is virtually confined to the second stage, antecedent events are often highly relevant. With the notable exception of breech presentation, serious injury to the child is almost always associated with outside intervention to effect delivery by traction because the mother is unable, unwilling or simply not given the opportunity to deliver herself.

Such was the emphasis placed on full dilatation in times past that it became generally accepted as the natural line of division between abdominal and vaginal delivery. This is a serious error fraught with the gravest consequences. In practical terms the second stage of labour is composed of two quite distinct phases. The first phase extends from full dilatation until the baby's head reaches the pelvic floor, and the second phase from then until the baby is born. These are as different as chalk is from cheese. The second stage, in other words, is not a single entity.

Phase One

During phase one of the second stage of labour the baby's head is high in the pelvis, the occiput is transverse, the vagina is not stretched and there is no inclination on the part of the mother to push. Neither the mother nor her attendants are aware of any change and the fact that the cervix has reached full dilatation would pass without notice unless, perchance, a pelvic examination is performed at this juncture. This phase is but a natural extension of the first stage of labour and treatment should not differ in any respect. A woman with no inclination to push should not be urged to do so. No attempt should be made to achieve vaginal delivery by traction with forceps and when the need for urgent delivery arises this should be by caesarean section. In terms of management, therefore, full dilatation of the cervix is an event of academic interest only. This reservation also applies to the time factor, a subject that is discussed in the following paragraph.

36

Phase Two

Phase two of the second stage of labour begins when the baby's head reaches the floor of the pelvis, an event that coincides with a dramatic change in the demeanor of the mother. Vaginal delivery is almost assured at this point and when the need for intervention arises the standard obstetric forceps can be used. The duration of this phase must be restricted because of the exceptional strain to which both mother and child are subjected by the compulsive desire to push. This is where the time factor becomes a vital consideration. There is no corresponding need to restrict the duration of phase one, where the element of exceptional strain does not operate.

Perhaps the most dangerous misunderstandings in current obstetric practice stem from a failure to clarify the distinction between the two phases of the second stage of labour. The classic example is when forceps are applied as a matter of course simply because the cervix is known to have been fully dilatated for an arbitrary period of time. A difficult rotation followed by strong traction leads to a diagnosis of cephalopelvic disproportion where none exists. The mother is exposed to the immediate risk of serious injury and her future plans are prejudiced by commital to elective caesarean section on the basis of wrong interpretation of the sequence of events. Furthermore, should the child die and necropsy show evidence of trauma, or alternatively should it survive with brain damage, this too is misinterpreted as further confirmation of the presence of cephalopelvic disproportion.

Forceps

The conventional method of treatment of slow progress in the second stage of labour is forceps extraction. Forceps are applied in three clinical circumstances which are quite different from one another, as follows.

First, the instrument may be applied as soon as full dilatation is achieved at the end of a long first stage of labour. The declared purpose is to bring the mother's ordeal to a speedy conclusion or to relieve fetal distress based sometimes on slender evidence. This is phase one of the second stage. The baby's head is still high and in the transverse diameter of the pelvis. Delivery entails rotation, frequently with Kielland's forceps, and considerable traction to overcome soft-part resistance because although the cervix is sufficiently dilatated, the vagina is most certainly not. This manoeuvre is the main source of serious injury to both mother and child in contemporary obstetrics. Perpetuation of the manoeuvre is based on the archaic proposition that full dilatation of the cervix is the natural line of demarcation between abdominal and vaginal delivery. This situation must change. It must be recognized that a case of this nature would fare much better if full dilatation were never achieved. At least this would protect against misguided attempts at vaginal delivery. It hardly needs to be said that the use of forceps, or ventouse, during the first stage of labour is indefensible in all circumstances.

Second, the instrument may be applied when uterine action fails as a secondary phenomenon after a relatively short first stage of labour. The baby's head remains high in the transverse position because the driving force is inadequate. From the point of view of vaginal delivery the prospect is the same, because the case remains in phase one of the second stage of labour.

Third, the instrument may be applied after the baby's head has reached the floor of the pelvis, when, despite good uterine action, the mother is unable to overcome the formidable obstacle presented by the levator muscles through her own efforts. Not infrequently this impasse arises because the mother is physically exhausted by a long first stage or is mentally confused by a large dose of drugs. She has, however, made the critical transition from phase one to phase two of the second stage of labour and extraction with forceps is now a comparatively safe procedure. The vagina, as well as the cervix, is fully dilated at this time.

Oxytocin as an Alternative

Conventional methods of treatment in phase one of the second stage of labour offer a straight choice between caesarean section and difficult forceps delivery. Faced with this choice, preference should always be for caesarean section, in the best interest of both parties.

There is, however, a third option: oxytocin. The relatively common clinical problem described above provides one of the most impressive examples of the intelligent use of oxytocin in the whole of obstetrics. An oxytocin infusion begun in the second stage of labour restores normal uterine action. This causes the baby's head to descend to the pelvic floor and hopefully also to rotate at that level. The result is a difficult rotational forceps delivery translated into an easy extraction, if not a spontaneous delivery. There is no better illustration of one of the basic concepts of Active Management of Labour: that delivery by propulsion is almost always preferable to delivery by traction. The use of oxytocin in the second stage of labour has made an important contribution to the reduction in the incidence of trauma to both mothers and infants in recent years, as illustrated in Table 5 and Graph 17.

Summary

Full dilatation of the cervix is certainly not the natural line of division between abdominal and vaginal delivery. The second stage of labour is composed of two distinct phases. The natural line of division between abdominal and vaginal delivery comes at the end of phase one, when the baby's head has descended to the floor of the pelvis, at which level rotation occurs. Vaginal delivery with forceps, or ventouse, should not be attempted simply because the case is in the second stage. Not only the cervix but also the vagina needs to be fully dilated. Kielland's forceps and the ventouse have both been discarded from this hospital, with no consequent increase in the rate of caesarean section. The explanation lies, at least in part, in the use of oxytocin during the second stage. This represents an important advance in the management of labour, particularly where trauma is concerned.

8

Acceleration of Slow Labour

The most important decisions relating to the management of labour are made during the first three hours. The decision to accelerate is one of these. Three hours after admission to a delivery unit the course of labour should be set to the extent that it should then be possible to predict the approximate time of delivery in all but a few instances. The ability to predict the time of delivery at this early stage is of inestimable value to all concerned.

Procedure

Circumstances dictate that the decision to accelerate progress—like the diagnosis of labour—must be made by a nurse, because nurses, unlike doctors, are physically present in a delivery unit at all times. Crucial decisions on management must not be allowed go by default simply because women admit themselves in labour at inconvenient hours. The duty of the consultant obstetrician is to clearly state the basic rules of procedure and this should entail accepting responsibility for the outcome. Prolonged labour has been virtually eliminated from this hospital mainly because the sister in charge of the delivery unit knows what to do and when to do it. She knows too that no blame will attach to her in the event of mishap. This is a vital consideration, without which no plan of action is likely to succeed. The procedure is as outlined below.

First assessment

Progress is assessed for the first time at one hour after admission. Artificial rupture of membranes is now performed. Apart from the fact that the nature of the liquor provides vital evidence of the fetal condition and therefore should be known in every case, there are four additional reasons why the membranes are ruptured at this time:

1. Rupture of membranes alone may be sufficient to accelerate in the event of slow progress (Graph 18).
2. Oxytocin is never used unless clear liquor is seen.
3. Oxytocin is often ineffective with intact membranes.
4. Theoretically at least, oxytocin may increase the risk of amniotic fluid infusion into the maternal circulation unless free drainage has been established.

39

Spontaneous rupture of membranes has already occurred in some 30% of women admitted to this hospital in labour.

Second assessment

Progress is assessed for the second time at two hours after admission. An oxytocin infusion is started unless significant progress—one notional centimetre at least—has been made since the previous examination. The decision to use oxytocin is taken by the sister in charge, without reference to medical staff. The following conditions must be fulfilled:

1. The mother must be a primigravida.
2. The presentation must be vertex.
3. The fetus must be single.
4. The membranes must be ruptured and clear liquor seen.

Oxytocin is prohibited in multigravidae, in malpresentations and twins, when membranes are intact or when meconium or no liquor is seen. The reasons for these exclusions are discussed elsewhere. Special attention is drawn to the fact that oxytocin may not be given to a parous woman without authorization in each individual case by a senior member of the medical staff, who must assume direct personal responsibility from this point. The decision to give oxytocin to a parous woman cannot be taken by a nurse or by a junior doctor.

Third assessment

Progress is assessed for the third time at three hours after admission. A dramatic change is expected. At this juncture it should be possible to predict full dilatation and consequently delivery from a straight projection on the partograph (Graph 11).

Subsequent assessments

Subsequent progress is assessed at intervals not exceeding two hours. In practice, the next examination is likely to be performed to confirm full dilatation because the mother feels the urge to push.

This makes a total of five pelvic examinations in the average case: at admission, to confirm the diagnosis of labour; at one, two and three hours, to monitor progress; and, finally, before the mother is allowed to push.

Slow Progress

In the event of failure to respond to treatment with oxytocin for a period of one hour, there are two possible explanations which should be considered. First, the woman may not be in labour because the initial diagnosis was wrong. Second, the forewaters may be intact despite the fact that liquor was seen to drain. Here again acceleration must not be confused with induction, where oxytocin frequently fails (Graphs 21 and 22).

Slow progress in labour is usually confined to women in whom the cervix is less than 2 cm dilated at the time of admission. When the cervix is more than 2 cm dilated at the time of admission there are few problems to be faced, diagnosis is easy, progress is rapid and delivery takes place within a matter of hours. The extent to which the cervix is dilated at the time of admission is an accurate reflection of the quality of uterine action and, contrary to widespread opinion, bears little if any relationship to the number of hours a woman has spent in labour at home. Forty per cent of primigravidae are delivered within four hours of admission to this hospital without treatment to accelerate progress (Table 8).

Secondary Arrest

In the event of secondary arrest in progress during the first stage of labour, when dilatation has been satisfactory in the early hours but comes to a virtual halt later, the same procedure is followed. Oxytocin is infused in the same manner. Caesarean section is undertaken after one hour, unless normal progress has resumed. This unusual pattern of dilatation raises the question of cephalopelvic disproportion and the diagnosis is confirmed should the pattern persist after good uterine action has been restored. Secondary arrest in progress may not occur until the second stage of labour has been reached, when, after full dilatation, the baby's head does not descend. Failure of descent is the clinical manifestation of dystocia during the second stage of labour and this should be seen as the counterpart of failure of the cervix to dilate during the first stage. The same procedure is followed. Oxytocin is infused (Graph 24). The second stage of labour is discussed in Chapter 7.

Summary

Duration of labour is determined by rate of dilatation of the cervix, especially during the early hours. Therefore it is essential that dilatation be recorded during this critical period. This requires pelvic examination at regular intervals for the first three hours. A nurse is the only person in a position to conduct regular examinations around the clock and to make the decision to accelerate when progress is slow. To meet this commitment, she must have precise instructions and must enjoy the unqualified support of her medical colleagues. The uterus in labour is almost uniformly responsive to oxytocin, provided the forewaters are ruptured. Oxytocin should not be given to parous women without authorization at the highest medical level in each case.

9

Oxytocin in Labour

Oxytocin is one of the most specific therapeutic agents available in medicine. Properly used it can also be one of the safest. The therapeutic effect of oxytocin is to cause the cervix to dilate during the first stage of labour and the baby's head to descend during the second stage. This sequential effect is almost invariably achieved. Indeed, the effect of oxytocin is so predictable that when the cervix does not dilate, during the first stage, far the most likely explanation is that the woman is not in labour. Failure of the cervix to dilate in response to oxytocin constitutes a clear indication to review the diagnosis of labour. And here it is necessary to re-emphasize the essential difference between induction of labour and acceleration of labour, because oxytocin is not nearly as predictable in initiating the process as it is in accelerating progress when labour has already started.

Explicit Rules

The rules that govern the use of oxytocin in this hospital are quite explicit and are rigidly enforced. Extensive practical experience has shown that these rules provide a very effective series of safeguards:

1. A standard concentration of 10 units of oxytocin in 1 litre of dextrose solution is used in all circumstances.
2. The total dose of oxytocin may not exceed 10 units.
3. The rate of infusion may not exceed 60 drops.*

Infusion of one litre at the rate prescribed imposes a time limit of six hours. This acts as an additional safety factor.

The only variable factor allowed is the rate of infusion. This begins at ten drops and increases by ten drops at intervals of 15 minutes to a maximum of 60 drops. The rate of infusion attains the maximum level of 60 drops in the shortest time, which is 75 minutes, in almost every instance. Evidence of fetal distress is the only absolute bar to this step-by-step method of progression (Graph 19).

---

*The drip set used conforms with the British Standard specification, which requires that 15–20 drops are equivalent to 1 ml. The maximun dose of oxytocin at 60 drops, therefore, is 40 milliunits per minute.

Hypertonic Uterine Action

The personal nurse—who accompanies every woman in labour—records each contraction as it occurs. The reverse side of the partograph is used for this purpose. The record is divided into periods of 15 minutes. The optimum number of contractions lies between five and seven. To guard against hypertonus, the number of contractions is not permitted to exceed seven in 15 minutes. Care is taken to ensure that the patient does not control the drip. This occurs, in practice, when the nurse reduces the rate of infusion simply because her patient complains of pain, which is of course only to be expected. This is a common manifestation of a low level of confidence in the system, which usually stems from imprecise instructions.

Special Equipment

No special equipment is used, either to dispense the oxytocin or to monitor its effects. Oxytocin is dispensed from a simple gravity feed regulated by the nurse. There is no inherent objection to automation provided that it does not become a mechanical substitute for individual attention. But it is a mistake to think that a precise dose of oxytocin in milliunits offers any material advantage. This is an item of utmost practical importance in centres where special equipment is not available.

The contribution of a personal nurse to a woman in labour extends far beyond supervision of oxytocin in the relatively few cases where this is given, while the answer to the suggestion, not infrequently made, that it is not feasible to provide personal attention on such a scale, is to remind the reader that this practice emanates from a large unit with some 8000 births per annum.

Causes of Confusion

The position with regard to oxytocin in some centres is indeed difficult to comprehend. There are several consultants, each with a fixed preference for a different regimen for which there is no factual basis. Intuitively, it seems, one feels that 2.5 units of oxytocin is best, another five units and another ten units, and to confuse the matter further some use all three consecutively in the same patient! This bizarre example of therapeutics, in which the dose of a drug is altered both in concentration and in rate of administration, can have few counterparts in any medical speciality. Is it any wonder that nurses called on to supervise similar patients in adjoining beds prescribed different concentrations of the same drug to treat the same disease, should feel confused? And when these complexities are compounded by ominous references to possible cephalopelvic disproportion, rupture of the uterus and injury to the child, their position becomes virtually untenable. The only sensible course open to a rational being placed in this position is to reduce the rate of infusion to an ineffectual level which is not sufficient to dilate the cervix, and to record hypertonic uterine action or fetal distress as the reason for doing so. This is what frequently happens in practice, thus giving rise to the mistaken impression that oxytocin is sometimes not an effective method of resolving the problem of slow labour. Nurses in this hospital are indemnified against the possibility of cephalopelvic disproportion, rupture of the uterus or injury to the child. Care is taken not to mention these subjects in the present context. Rather, criticism is reserved for those who fail to act promptly to limit the duration of labour.

Water Intoxication

The only direct toxic effect of oxytocin is water intoxication. This classic syndrome—which may result in convulsions, coma and even death—is due to an intrinsic antidiuretic effect of oxytocin which results in reabsorption of salt-free water from the renal tubules. As its name implies, water intoxication is directly related to the volume of fluid available. The possibility of water intoxication arises when more than 3 litres of salt-free fluid are administered by the intravenous route. This cannot happen when the rules previously stated are followed. The fact that the volume of fluid is restricted to 1 litre provides an absolute guarantee against water intoxication. Naturally, notice must also be taken of other sources of fluid given intravenously, as for example, by an anaesthetist in conjunction with an epidural block. This can be an important source of additional fluid, especially when epidural block is misused as a cover for prolonged labour. The longer the labour, the greater the volume of fluid infused. Oral fluids do not contribute to water intoxication because they are regulated by the patient herself, not forced upon her.

Water intoxication is much more likely to occur when oxytocin is used to induce labour, because induction is too often allowed to continue for an indefinite period of time, during which a very considerable volume of salt-free fluid may be infused.

Neonatal Jaundice

An association between oxytocin and neonatal jaundice has attracted attention in recent years. Studies in this hospital have confirmed that there is an overall increase in the incidence of neonatal jaundice in cases treated with oxytocin, but they have also shown that this increase is confined to cases in which oxytocin is used to induce labour. There is no increase in cases in which oxytocin is used to accelerate labour already started. The overall increase in the incidence of neonatal jaundice associated with oxytocin is therefore a product of the relative state of immaturity that results from interruption of the course of pregnancy before the natural conclusion; it is not a direct toxic effect of oxytocin. This constitutes yet another example of the need to draw a distinction between induction and acceleration[10].

Trauma

For many years it has been taught that oxytocin increases the risk of trauma to both mother and child, especially where there is an element of cephalopelvic disproportion. There is no foundation for this suggestion, at least in primigravidae. In primigravidae the opposite is the case because efficient uterine action reduces the need for traction, which is the real cause of trauma. There was no case of rupture of the uterus in some 50 000 consecutive primigravidae delivered in this hospital during the 20-odd years under review. Neither was there a case of traumatic intracranial haemorrhage, in a cephalic presentation, that was not delivered with forceps. The incidence of traumatic intracranial haemorrhage in cephalic presentations showed a sharp decline after the present policy of prevention of prolonged labour was introduced. The fundamental difference between primigravidae and multigravidae must be noted once more because oxytocin is surely a potent cause of rupture of the uterus in parous women. The subject of trauma is dealt with at length in Chapter 14.

Hypoxia

Hypoxia is a different proposition. Every contraction of the uterus reduces circulation through the placenta, even during the course of normal labour. This presents no serious problem to a fetus who starts labour with a normal placenta, but it can have grave consequences should placental function already be impaired. A fetus with normal placental function is well equipped to withstand the stress of normal labour unless an accident such as prolapse of the cord should occur. The fetus who suffers from hypoxia during the course of normal labour is the fetus whose placental function is impaired before labour began. To the fetus, the consequences are the same whether the natural action of the uterus is sufficient to dilate the cervix or inefficient uterine action is corrected with oxytocin. Since the purpose of oxytocin is to stimulate normal uterine action it follows that circulation through the placenta must be reduced; and in this sense it is inevitable that oxytocin should contribute to the problem of hypoxia. This is not a direct toxic effect of oxytocin but a by-product of efficient uterine action.

Summary

Oxytocin is an extraordinarily effective preparation for the treatment of slow labour, but strict rules are necessary to ensure that it is properly used. Its use should be confined to primigravidae with malpresentations, hydrocephalus and twins specifically excluded. The dose should not exceed 10 units, the volume 1 litre and the rate 60 drops per minute. There should be a time limit of six hours. Subject to these restrictions, fetal hypoxia is the only problem. Oxytocin should never be used when there is evidence of impaired placental function or fetal distress. Water intoxication should never occur.

10

Normal and Abnormal Labour (Dystocia)

It may well seem strange that the parameters of normal labour to which all concerned with management should consciously aspire are seldom if ever defined. Although the result is unlikely to gain universal acceptance in every last detail, this is an immensely rewarding exercise. A clear definition of normal labour should be posted in a prominent position in every delivery unit—and every classroom—to serve as a statement of common purpose. The subject should be considered in broad outline, with minor detail best avoided.

In this hospital labour is classified as normal when a baby is born through the natural passages, by the efforts of the mother, within a reasonable time span, and no harm befalls either party as a result of the experience. Twelve hours is regarded as a reasonable time span.

Conversely, labour is classified as abnormal when delivery is by caesarean section or through the natural passages by the efforts of the doctor, when duration exceeds 12 hours, or when some harm befalls either party.

A priori, the induction of labour is designated abnormal, as are all operative deliveries. This is not to say that induction, caesarean section and low forceps are not practised, but rather that they are practised with discretion and always as the lesser of two evils. Neither Kielland's forceps nor ventouse are used.

Although at first sight these definitions may appear somewhat unrealistic to those accustomed to think of childbirth in terms of operative procedures, developments in this hospital over the past 20 years have shown that this viewpoint is not now tenable.

Abnormal labour has three possible causes: inefficient uterine action, occipitoposterior position and cephalopelvic disproportion. These three correspond with faults in the passage, faults in the passenger and faults in the forces, but, significantly, the order of priority is reversed. Attention is again directed to the fact that the term cephalopelvic disproportion as used throughout this manual refers only to primigravidae and, furthermore, that malpresentations, and malformations, are not included under this heading. Malpresentations, and malformations, are the subject of a separate chapter; these may cause the syndrome of obstructed labour, which constitutes a different clinical problem altogether.

There is bound to be some subjective element in the differential diagnosis between the three possible causes of abnormal labour in individual cases.

46

Occipitoposterior position is the exception because in a negative sense, at least, it can be excluded at pelvic examination. The main problem lies between inefficient uterine action and cephalopelvic disproportion. The differential diagnosis between these two is based largely on personal intuition. Local custom frequently determines which cases of abnormal labour are attributed to cephalopelvic disproportion, while X-ray pelvimetries are used to bolster opinions that are preconceived. This practice is very evident in the wide variation in recorded incidence of cephalopelvic disproportion in the Annual Clinical Reports of maternity hospitals that are located in the same geographical region and which appear similar in all other respects. The recorded incidence of cephalopelvic disproportion is merely a statement of the number of caesarean sections arbitrarily included under this classification. This is an implausible method of estimating the true prevalence of a disease and obviously one on which no reliance can be placed.

Traditionally, cephalopelvic disproportion has been taught to medical students and pupil midwives as the most important cause of abnormal labour. Possibly this arose out of concern that serious harm might befall both mother and child should the condition be overlooked. This is a fundamental mistake, for which there is absolutely no clinical evidence. There can be little doubt that the error arose because cephalopelvic disproportion in primigravidae and obstructed labour in multigravidae were not recognized as entirely different clinical entities, with different causes, different treatments and different results. Even more important in this regard was the failure to recognize that the primigravid uterus is virtually immune to rupture, whereas the multigravid uterus is rupture-prone.

Probably the most significant outcome of Active Management of Labour is that effective uterine action is assured in every case, with the result that the problem of cephalopelvic disproportion has been isolated for the first time. The differential diagnosis between inefficient uterine action, cephalopelvic disproportion and occipitoposterior position can now be made by a simple process of exclusion. Given a cervix that dilates progressively and an occiput not posterior, a diagnosis of cephalopelvic disproportion can confidently be made.

The causes of abnormal labour are discussed in Chapters 11, 12 and 13, and these should be read in conjunction with this chapter.

Summary

Far too much time and attention is devoted to consideration of abnormal labour and to how to surmount the problems by surgical means without first defining the norm to which all should aspire.

11

Inefficient Uterine Action

Inefficient uterine action is far and away the most common complication of labour in primigravidae. This is certainly not so in multigravidae. A diagnosis of inefficient uterine action in a multigravida should always be viewed with the gravest suspicion because the parous uterus is by nature a highly efficient organ with much less resistance to overcome. Slow progress in a multigravida may well be an expression of obstruction and obstructed labour in a multigravida is much the commonest cause of rupture of the uterus. Essential differences between primigravid and multigravid labour need constant reiteration. The present chapter on inefficient uterine action refers to *primigravidae* only; the contents should be applied to multigravidae with extreme caution.

Definitions

The sole function of the uterus during the first stage of labour is to cause the cervix to dilate, while during the second stage of labour it is to cause the baby's head to descend to the level of the pelvic floor. These separate functions must not be confused. Pressure on the pelvic floor activates the reflex action of voluntary muscles, which in turn cause the baby to be born. The efficiency of the uterus during labour can be gauged only by its ability to complete these specific functions, each within a reasonable period of time. In other words the efficiency of the uterus can be measured only in terms of the results achieved. These results correlate equally poorly with the subjective sensation of pain as felt by the mother or with the objective assessment of contractions made by the attendant. Success or failure of treatment of inefficient uterine action must be evaluated in a similar fashion.

Acceptance of Oxytocin

Although the means, in the form of oxytocin, have long been available, systematic treatment of inefficient uterine action has been slow to develop. The reasons for this delay seem to have been as follows:

1. Since the first step towards the solution of a problem is accurate definition, failure to submit the syndrome of abnormal labour to detailed analysis rendered any solution virtually impossible.

2. Inefficient uterine action, which is by far the most common cause of abnormal labour, was itself complicated by being subdivided into two distinct types, described as hypotonic and hypertonic inertia. This subdivision was coupled with the warning that although stimulation with oxytocin could be beneficial to the former, it could be detrimental to the latter. There is no basis for this assertion in practice; inefficient uterine action is a single clinical entity which is uniformly responsive to stimulation with oxytocin.

3. The treatment of inefficient uterine action was further inhibited by the proposition, which amounted to almost an article of faith, that stimulation of the uterus in circumstances in which there was even the faintest possibility of cephalopelvic disproportion could result in serious injury to both mother and child. As, strictly speaking, cephalopelvic disproportion can never be wholly excluded until labour has come to a successful conclusion, this caveat ensured that oxytocin could not be used to proper effect for fear of dire consequences. As labour could not be brought to a successful conclusion without efficient uterine action, this was a classic example of the chicken and egg situation. The result was therapeutic paralysis.

Clinical Types

Typically, inefficient uterine action presents as slow dilatation of the cervix, which continues from the very onset of labour. This persistent pattern of slow dilatation should lead to an early diagnosis and prompt treatment, long before dehydration, ketosis and other evidence of physical or mental exhaustion make their appearance. The cervix of a woman in labour is so predictably responsive to stimulation with oxytocin that when the rate of dilatation does not accelerate sharply, the initial diagnosis of labour is almost certainly wrong. Where little attention is paid to the diagnosis of labour such cases are commonplace and may soon create the impression that oxytocin is not an altogether reliable method of treatment. Otherwise this false impression may derive from the widespread confusion between acceleration and induction, where there is of course no clear indication as to when labour begins. It is of the utmost importance to appreciate that slow dilatation of the cervix as a primary phenomenon is not at all suggestive of cephalopelvic disproportion, or of its clinical counterpart, occipitoposterior position.

Less frequently, inefficient uterine action develops as a secondary phenomenon, presenting as an arrest in dilatation of the cervix late in the first stage of labour, after there has been a normal start. Secondary arrest in dilatation of the cervix is indeed suggestive of cephalopelvic disproportion, but because inefficient uterine action is still the commonest cause, cases should be treated with oxytocin for a limited period of time before resort is made to caesarean section for the alternative indications of cephalopelvic disproportion or occipitoposterior position.

Finally, inefficient uterine action may not develop until the second stage of labour, when it presents as failure of the baby's head to descend after full dilatation has been achieved. The clinical situation is the same as described in the previous paragraph and oxytocin should be given for a limited period of time before resort is made to caesarean section. Forcible vaginal delivery with forceps should not be undertaken at this juncture simply because the cervix has reached full dilatation (Graphs 13, 14, 15 and 16).

Summary

The outstanding lesson learned about labour in recent years is that efficient uterine action represents the key to normality and, furthermore, that efficient uterine action can be safely assured through the judicious use of oxytocin. There is, however, one important qualification: that a clear distinction be maintained between primigravidae and multigravidae at all times. The assurance of efficient uterine action in all primigravidae has had the effect of isolating the problem of cephalopelvic disproportion as a distinct entity for the very first time. The result has been a radical change in the whole approach to the management of labour.

12

Cephalopelvic Disproportion

The concept of cephalopelvic disproportion has coloured attitudes to labour for a very long time[3]. The main reason for this is that cephalopelvic disproportion is coupled in the collective subconscious of obstetricians with the threat of rupture of the uterus and trauma to the child. Hence it comes as no little surprise to learn that in the whole of recorded clinical experience there is no factual basis whatever for either contention. Of course this is to presume that the term 'cephalopelvic disproportion' is used correctly to refer to primigravidae only and not extended incorrectly to include multigravidae also. Rupture of the uterus is a calamity that befalls multigravidae with obstructed labour, usually caused by mal-presentations. It does not affect primigravidae with cephalopelvic disproportion. Moreover, trauma to the child is almost exclusively associated with instrumental delivery. The subject of trauma is discussed at greater length in Chapter 14.

There may have been good reason for the widespread concern about cephalopelvic disproportion when rickets was a common disease. But this situation no longer exists. In retrospect, it now seems to have been an unfortunate coincidence that X-ray pelvimetry was perfected at the same time as the social conditions that gave rise to rickets were eradicated, more than a generation ago. This has served to perpetuate a preoccupation with a condition that nowadays is hardly ever seen. At the time X-ray pelvimetry seemed to provide an objective scientific basis for the study of cephalopelvic disproportion because it reduced the issue to a simple question of shape and size—items that could be accurately portrayed. A diagnosis of contracted pelvis, and by inference cephalopelvic disproportion, was compared with an orthopaedic fracture: a straightforward matter of modern equipment and technical expertise. It seemed all too reasonable to conclude that accurate measurements of the pelvis could only be helpful to a woman facing labour for the first time, as it would have seemed perverse to suggest that such measurements could, in the event, be a liability. But this has in fact proved to be the case.

The procedure in those days was to combine digital assessment of the pelvis with a head-fitting test, sometimes under general anaesthesia, in every primigravida in whom the baby's head had not engaged at, say, 38 weeks. This was combined with X-ray pelvimetry. Then a choice was made between delivery by elective caesarean section and trial of labour. Frequently this crucial decision, which could have permanent effects on a woman's lifestyle, was made, albeit indirectly, by a radiologist who had never seen the patient.

Childbirth was governed by architectural nuances.

A trial of labour was carefully documented in advance. Antenatal notes included predictions that were usually pessimistic and almost always cautionary in tone. Nowhere was it appreciated that a trial of labour might fail simply because the outcome was prejudiced beforehand or because an intolerable burden of responsibility was placed on nurses and resident doctors by these reservations, so freely expressed by their senior colleagues. There was an absolute bar on the use of oxytocin because it was taken for granted that stimulation of the uterus in the presence of suspected cephalopelvic disproportion could easily result in serious injury to mother or child. Furthermore, when the uterus did not act effectively to dilate the cervix, this was seen as a protective mechanism, which served only to confirm the original suspicion. Finally, a diagnosis of cephalopelvic disproportion once made was, in effect, permanent, so that later children were delivered by elective caesarean section, without further consideration. This method of procedure had important long-term implications for the woman and her family, which attracted surprisingly little attention.

Ironically it was in this hospital that the operation of symphysiotomy was revived in the 1940s to offset this commitment to repeat caesarean sections in young mothers with a diagnosis of cephalopelvic disproportion. This practice continued for 20 years until Active Management of Labour, which ensured efficient uterine action for every woman in labour, was introduced in the 1960s. It soon became apparent that most women previously treated by symphysiotomy or caesarean section suffered not from cephalopelvic disproportion but from inefficient uterine action. Within a few years the recorded incidence of cephalopelvic disproportion had fallen to a small fraction of the previous level.

Definition

'Cephalopelvic disproportion' is a term used only in the context of first-time mothers with normal cephalic presentations. The restricted use of the term is considered a matter of fundamental importance. The term is advisedly not used in the context of subsequent births, nor does it include malpresentations or hydrocephalus, whatever the mother's parity. 'Obstructed labour' is a term used to describe a completely different clinical entity which involves the fetus directly, such as brow or shoulder presentation, or hydrocephalus. Here the capacity of the pelvis is not the real issue. Obstructed labour, in particular in a multigravida, is a much more serious proposition than cephalopelvic disproportion (in a primigravida), because it is all too likely to lead to rupture of the uterus. Rupture of the uterus becomes almost inevitable should the condition escape notice and oxytocin be infused to stimulate an organ that is efficient by nature. The altogether mistaken belief that a similar fate might befall a primigravida with cephalopelvic disproportion, or indeed obstruction, stems from a failure to draw a clear distinction between mothers on the grounds of parity.

Diagnosis

No consideration whatsoever is given to the possibility of cephalopelvic disproportion in the course of routine antenatal care at this hospital. All reference to the subject is consciously excluded. No mention is made in case notes, in the firm belief that this has an adverse effect on the eventual outcome. The pelvis is not assessed by clinical means, nor is X-ray pelvimetry undertaken. The result is that elective caesarean section is never performed for this indication. And, in particular, the term 'trial of labour' is studiously avoided.

The possibility of cephalopelvic disproportion is raised for the very first time when the course of labour proves abnormal. Abnormal labour becomes evident when the cervix fails to dilate progressively during the first stage or the baby's head fails to descend during the second stage. Slow progress as a primary event, that is early in labour, is always considered an expression of inefficient uterine action, whereas slow progress as a secondary event, late in labour, is at least sometimes considered an expression of cephalopelvic disproportion. Nevertheless, a diagnosis of cephalopelvic disproportion is not seriously entertained until oxytocin has been infused for a reasonable period of time to eliminate inefficient uterine action, which remains a much more likely cause even of this type of secondary arrest. A tentative diagnosis of cephalopelvic disproportion is made when progress remains unsatisfactory— provided that the occiput is not posterior. These are the clinical circumstances in which caesarean section for cephalopelvic disproportion is performed. No attempt is made to anticipate these events because such attempts have led us to much unnecessary intervention in previous years (Graph 24).

Even so, the final decision is postponed until the puerperium when, for the purpose of medical records, every case of abnormal labour is reviewed. A differential diagnosis between inefficient uterine action, cephalopelvic disproportion and occipitoposterior position is made in the light of all the evidence available after the event. X-ray pelvimetry may be requested at this stage mainly, it must be said, as an academic exercise. This final decision, which is recorded on the woman's case notes, strongly influences the mode of delivery on the next occasion.

Again for the purpose of medical records, a diagnosis of cephalopelvic disproportion is positively excluded in every case in which labour is classified as normal because vaginal delivery has been achieved within 12 hours and there has been no significant injury to mother or child. This means that a decision for or against a diagnosis of cephalopelvic disproportion is made in every primigravida delivered. The recorded incidence of cephalopelvic disproportion based on this method of selection has remained at approximately one in 250 primigravidae for the past 20 years. Yet in spite of this very low figure, one in every two cases in which a diagnosis of cephalopelvic disproportion was made subsequently had a vaginal delivery. Cephalopelvic disproportion therefore is clearly not a common disorder.

Pelvic Deformity

Pelvic deformity is considered a separate entity. Less than one in every thousand women is affected in this way. Almost invariably the deformity is caused either by a limp in childhood or by a crush injury in adult life. Diagnosis presents no problem; cases declare themselves in the patient's gait or in the history of a road traffic accident. In this hospital these are virtually the only cases delivered by elective caesarean section for reasons of pelvic architecture.

Change in Practice

In recent years no single aspect of obstetric practice in this hospital has undergone such radical change as cephalopelvic disproportion. The change has come about as a result of a combination of factors, chief amongst which are: insistence on the precise use of terms, realization that uterine action is the key to normal birth, and conclusive evidence that oxytocin can be used safely in primigravidae. Now it has become abundantly clear that all attempts at diagnosis of cephalopelvic disproportion beforehand are misguided because they result in a rate of intervention grossly in excess of the true prevalence of the disorder. This represents a classic example of a situation in which the application of the laudable principle of prevention becomes counterproductive in its effects. Hence the term 'trial of labour' has been deleted from our vocabulary, while antenatal X-ray pelvimetry is no longer practised. Not even stature is regarded as of much significance, because small mothers have small babies. This generalization seems to have global significance, as for example in Asia and Africa, where Western observers tend to place undue emphasis on short stature, without directing equal attention to low birth weight.

Summary

The term 'cephalopelvic disproportion' applies only to primigravidae. Furthermore, malpresentations, and malformations, are specifically excluded from consideration under this heading. The approach is entirely pragmatic and a prospective diagnosis is never made. The possibility of cephalopelvic disproportion is first mooted when labour ceases to progress, but a diagnosis is not considered unless efficient uterine action has been assured for a reasonable period of time. This requires oxytocin, which can be given in the sure knowledge that it does not rupture the primigravid uterus or cause trauma to the child. Therefore, whereas others say 'don't use oxytocin unless cephalopelvic disproportion has been excluded' we say 'cephalopelvic disproportion cannot be excluded unless oxytocin is used'.

13

Occipitoposterior Position

Occipitoposterior position is the third and only other possible cause of abnormal labour. The clinical problems posed are very similar to those of cephalopelvic disproportion. But there is one important difference: it is quite a simple matter to determine the position of the occiput by pelvic examination. Diagnosis in this sense is a straightforward procedure.[7]

Management

The same pragmatic approach is adopted to occipitoposterior position as to cephalopelvic disproportion. No attention is paid to the matter during the later weeks of pregnancy, and to avoid giving rise to the impression that position may have an adverse effect on the subsequent course of labour, no record is made at antenatal clinics. As with cephalopelvic disproportion, the greater the emphasis, the more likely it is that difficulties will follow. The anxious doctor creates his own problems under these headings.

The question of occipitoposterior position does not arise until the course of labour has already proved abnormal. This is evident when the cervix fails to dilate during the first stage or the baby's head fails to descend during the second stage. Slow progress as a primary event, that is early in labour, is always considered an expression of inefficient uterine action, whereas slow progress as a secondary event, late in labour is sometimes considered an expression of cephalopelvic disproportion and sometimes of occipitoposterior position. But even then inefficient uterine action is still the most likely cause. Secondary arrest of progress late in labour which does not respond to stimulation with oxytocin after a reasonable period of time is attributed to malposition when the occiput is posterior and to cephalopelvic disproportion when this is not so. Caesarean section is performed in either event unless the cervix is fully dilated.

In practice the most dangerous aspect of occipitoposterior position emerges during the second stage of labour, when the temptation to opt for vaginal delivery seems almost irresistible. There are still too many obstetricians who equate full dilatation with the point of no return in labour, after which vaginal delivery becomes a challenge to manual dexterity. This attitude leads to forcible rotation and extraction with forceps—the manoeuvre that carries the greatest risk of trauma to both mother and child in contemporary obstetrics. In this hospital a case of occipitoposterior position that persists for more than one hour into the second stage of labour is delivered by caesarean section, without regard to the fact that the cervix is fully dilated, unless the baby's head is on the pelvic floor and manual rotation can be performed easily or vaginal delivery effected face to pubis. Forceps are never used to rotate, nor is the head displaced upwards for this purpose.

Transverse Arrest

The term 'transverse arrest' is widely misunderstood. The normal position of the occiput is in the transverse diameter of the pelvis until the baby's head reaches the level of the ischial spines, which mark the junction between the mid-strait and the outlet of the bony pelvis. The ischial spines also mark the level of transition between phase one and phase two of the second stage of labour, described in Chapter 7, because they provide the attachments of the levator ani muscles, which together form the floor of the pelvis. It is also at this level that the reflex action of voluntary muscles is activated and rotation of occiput normally occurs. Rotation is effected by the combined action of the uterus and voluntary muscles, and when it fails it is because this composite force is not equal to the task. Hence arrest in the transverse diameter of the pelvis is not, as the term implies, the result of physical obstruction but an expression of inadequate driving force. Transverse arrest is not the cause of delay but the result. Treatment of transverse arrest is therefore treatment of delay in the second stage. In the case of mid-transverse arrest, so named because the head is above the level of the ischial spines, oxytocin is used to improve the action of the uterus and so propel the head downwards to the level at which rotation normally occurs. In the case of deep transverse arrest, so named because the head is already at the level of the ischial spines, manual rotation and routine forceps extraction is permitted. No attempt is made to rotate and extract a head in the mid-strait of the pelvis; caesarean section is performed whenever the need for delivery arises in these circumstances.

The widespread misunderstanding that exists in respect of the significance of transverse arrest is reflected in the exaggerated attention paid to minor variations in the shape and size of the pelvis in centres where antenatal X-ray pelvimetry is practised. There is an unwarranted assumption that prominent ischial spines cause deep transverse arrest and long before labour even begins forecasts are made of likely trouble at the pelvic outlet. This is a characteristic feature of the mechanical approach to childbirth, in which the shape and size of the pelvis rather than the functional efficiency of the uterus is the main focus of attention.

Results

The position of the occiput has an adverse effect on the outcome of labour in approximately one in every 250 primigravidae delivered in this hospital. By coincidence this is the same as the figure quoted for cephalopelvic disproportion in Chapter 12. In effect, this means that eight in every 1000 primigravidae—less than 1%—do not achieve the goal of safe vaginal delivery within a reasonable period of time, as a result of either condition. The differential diagnosis is based more or less entirely on the position of the occiput at the point of delivery and is made in retrospect. Inevitably there is some degree of overlap, but this does not affect management.

Summary

There is a very close similarity between persistent occipitoposterior position and cephalopelvic disproportion in clinical practice. Particular care must be taken not to create problems under either heading by making predictions on the outcome of labour. As in cephalopelvic disproportion forecasts in this direction have a strong tendency to self-fulfilment. Occipitoposterior position should not be cited as the cause of abnormal labour until inefficient uterine action has been positively excluded, if need be with oxytocin. Although occipitoposterior position may result in slow progress late in the first stage of labour, the main danger arises early in the second stage, when there is a strong temptation to attempt vaginal delivery in unfavourable circumstances, before the head has descended to a safe level. The term 'transverse arrest' should be discarded completely as a misnomer based on a lack of understanding of the natural process of descent and rotation during the course of normal labour.

14

Trauma

Trauma in obstetrics should be considered as a single entity because the circumstances that give rise to it in the mother are the same as those that give rise to it in the child. These arise late in labour and are associated almost invariably with medical intervention at the point of delivery. Breech presentation is the exception: trauma in breech presentation is confined to the fetus and is inherent in the mode of birth.

Injury to the Mother

Rupture of the uterus is the classic example of serious trauma to the mother.[1] This catastrophe is not likely to escape notice because it entails massive blood transfusion, hysterectomy and even death. The first case reported in the medical literature in a primigravida and not associated with manipulation occurred in a woman who was treated with oxytocin under cover of epidural anaesthesia in the course of a labour that was allowed to continue for more than 50 hours (Daw, E. (1973) *Journal of Obstetrics and Gynaecology of the British Commonwealth*, 80: 374–375). This bizarre case hardly needs further comment and could be regarded as the exception that proves the rule enunciated in this manual: that the primigravid uterus is virtually immune to rupture, except by manipulation. There was, of course, no case of a ruptured uterus in almost 50 000 consecutive primigravidae delivered in this hospital during the period of 20 years under review, despite extensive use of oxytocin to accelerate progress in some 15 000 cases, in both the first and second stages of labour (see Table 4).

Laceration of the cervix, rupture of the vault and spiral tears of the vagina are somewhat less dramatic manifestations of serious trauma to the mother which also may entail profuse haemorrhage, blood transfusion and extensive surgical repair. Although not so easy to quantify in numerical terms, these injuries are likewise almost always associated with assisted delivery, especially when forceps are used for the purpose of rotation in phase one of the second stage of labour.

Injury to the Child

Rupture of tentorium cerebelli is the corresponding example of serious trauma to the child.[12] This lesion, which results in subdural haemorrhage, can be demonstrated at post-mortem examination and affords conclusive evidence of cause of death. It has a special association with breech presentation and this is one of the main reasons why all malpresentations are excluded from consideration in this manual. Equally important but not so well appreciated is the fact that virtually every case of injury to the tentorium that is not associated with breech presentation is associated with forceps delivery. There were 44 cases of traumatic intracranial haemorrhage in first-born infants delivered in this hospital during the period 1963–1979 inclusive: 27 were cephalic presentations, all of which were delivered with forceps. There was no case of traumatic intracranial haemorrhage other than in breech or forceps delivery. This statement is made possible only by the comprehensive post-mortem coverage during those years.

The close association between trauma in the mother and trauma in the child is well illustrated by the 27 cases of traumatic intracranial haemorrhage in cephalic presentations described in the previous paragraph. The results in these 27 mothers were as follows: one maternal death, eight blood transfusions for traumatic haemorrhage, one persistent foot-drop, and three mothers retained in hospital for more than two weeks—a total of 13 individual cases, or almost 50%.

Inexperience on the part of the doctor was not a factor in these cases, because the forceps were applied by a consultant in ten cases, by a senior resident in 14 cases and by a junior resident in only 3 cases. A clear association between trauma and duration is evident from the fact that labour was prolonged, more than 12 hours, in no less than 16 of the 27 cases.

Prevention of Trauma

A sharp decline in the incidence of trauma occurred after the decision was taken to limit the duration of labour to 12 hours. Meanwhile, although the manoeuvre of rotation with forceps was discarded, there was no increase in the number of caesarean sections performed. The explanation is that more babies were born by propulsion and fewer by traction, especially combined with rotation.

An anomaly in contemporary attitudes to the fetus in labour is evident in the contrast that exists between the high level of attention paid to hypoxia and the almost casual approach to trauma. A fetus supervised with great care throughout pregnancy and the first stage of labour is subjected to a degree of trauma at the point of delivery that would not be considered tolerable under any circumstances a few hours later. Forcible delivery is sometimes undertaken for no better reason than that the cervix is fully dilated for a specified time. At other times trauma is inflicted in the course of a frantic effort to rescue the fetus from a condition of distress based on very slender evidence. The doctor, understandably anxious to save the fetus from hypoxia, exposes it to trauma and introduces the risk of serious injury to the mother in the process. Death in these circumstances is almost sure to be attributed to hypoxia unless a post-mortem examination is performed, and even then it is often wrongly assumed that intracranial haemorrhage was the cause of the fetal distress rather than the result of treatment. The sequence of mistakes is complete when the traumatic intracranial haemorrhage is attributed to cephalopelvic disproportion. Cephalopelvic disproportion is positively not a significant factor in the aetiology of trauma. Fourteen of the 27 mothers referred to previously returned to this hospital for their second birth: 13 had a spontaneous delivery of a healthy infant which weighed more than the first in all but two instances. Furthermore, six of the 27 infants were preterm. This confirms the general belief that preterm infants are more vulnerable than term infants, but it is notable that the only preterm infants who died from traumatic intracranial haemorrhage were delivered with forceps. This points strongly to the conclusion that it was the forceps rather than the immaturity that was the decisive factor. Consequently, delivery of preterm infants with forceps is not to be recommended as a prophylactic measure against trauma.

Summary

Breech presentation apart, trauma in obstetrics is associated to an over-whelming degree with delivery by traction. Trauma is therefore much more common in primigravidae. The use of oxytocin to ensure efficient uterine action reduces the need for traction because it supports the natural process of propulsion that enables primigravidae to deliver themselves. Forceps do not protect the immature head from trauma, rather the opposite is the case.

15

Pain

The most characteristic feature of the conventional attitude to management of labour is the strong emphasis placed on the element of pain and consequently on drugs for the relief of pain. There are many delivery units that operate on the simple premise that virtually the only and certainly the most valuable contribution a nurse or doctor can make to the comfort of a woman in labour is to ensure that she receives analgesic agents in adequate amounts. This passive attitude to management has led to widespread abuse of drugs and the results are far from impressive even in the short-term sense of immediate consumer satisfaction. That there is a physical element in the pain of labour is not open to question, but it is equally true that the nature of the pain is patently different from the pain associated with surgical operations, or other forms of injury for which similar drugs are prescribed.[6]

First Stage

Pain during the first stage of labour is intermittent, lasts not longer than one minute, and then ceases completely. A woman can expect approximately five such pains in each period of 15 minutes, which makes a total of 100 pains during the course of a first labour of average duration. The pains occur somewhat less frequently at the beginning and more frequently at the end. The type of pain is a cramp comparable with primary spasmodic dysmenorrhoea, with which almost every woman is familiar.

The nature of the pain during the first stage of labour is quite different from that during the second stage. An important component of pain during the first stage derives from a mounting sense of frustration which a woman often endures because she feels herself to be a helpless victim of powerful natural forces over which she can exercise little or no influence. Swept along on a tide of events, the purpose of which she often does not comprehend, she tends to lose self-control. This is especially so when progress is slow and no one can say when her ordeal is likely to end. Meanwhile nurses come and go at regular intervals of eight hours, but for her the problem seems to begin all over again. For these reasons and because of the comparatively long duration, the problem of pain relief in labour is essentially a problem of the first stage, during the tedious hours while the cervix dilates. Acceleration with oxytocin is therefore often more constructive than analgesia in the relief of pain. A dramatic improvement in the outlook of a woman in labour can be expected when the impasse that results from inefficient uterine action is broken and progress is restored. This despite the fact that contractions are much stronger.

Second Stage

The nature of the pain during the second stage of labour is quite different from that during the first stage. Although the physical element of discomfort is much more in evidence during the second stage, a woman is better able to cope because she is actively involved. Now she senses that the end is near and furthermore that it can be hastened by her own efforts. She can regain control of the situation as the tremendous exertion involved in pushing distracts her attention from uterine contractions. A priori, it must be assumed that almost every mother wishes to give birth to her own child. Few mothers, irrespective of appearances at the time, wish the doctor to act as a surrogate.

Reaction to Pain

Women seem to react instinctively to the pain of labour. Initially startled, then tense, then restive and finally limp when, with closed eyes, they withdraw completely from contact with their surroundings. The intensity of the reaction grows with successive pains until it extends to fill the interval between contractions so that there is no longer any period of relaxation. This situation, in which a woman continues to react long after a contraction has passed, should not be allowed to develop, because, once lost, contact is seldom possible to restore. Loss of contact with a woman in labour is generally a product of poor management, to which analgesic drugs are not the answer.

But surely the most impressive feature of pain in labour is the extraordinary variation in the reaction of different persons to what is in effect the same stimulus. Although objective measurements indicate that uterine contractions are of similar frequency, similar strength and similar duration, the very wide range in the response of different individuals affords clear evidence of the paramount importance of the subjective element in the pain. Emotional stability is always put to the test in times of stress and there is no stress in the life of an average person, man or woman, to compare with the birth of a first child. Hence the whole spectrum of human behaviour is revealed in a busy delivery unit in the course of a single day. To concentrate on the physical element in the pain of labour to the virtual exclusion of the subjective response is comparable to concentrating on the virulence of the organism in the case of infection without due regard to the resistance of the host. In general terms, much more can be achieved through action taken to raise the level of resistance to pain that can be achieved by the use of analgesic drugs. This is also the human way because it leaves a mother in full control of her faculties, enhances her sense of dignity and permits her to deliver her own child. In an ideal world there would be no need for drugs to relieve pain in labour. Although this happy state may still appear far off to many, it should be noted that 50% of primigravidae delivered in this hospital receive no medication whatsoever. Apropos of this, the signal importance attached to duration of exposure and to continuous personal support throughout are discussed in Chapters 4 and 19.

No analgesic drug is ever given until a firm diagnosis of labour has been made and a woman is therefore committed to delivery. This is an absolute rule and evasions are not tolerated under the guise of ambivalent terms such as false or latent labour. The use of analgesic drugs on speculative grounds, to see what happens, is condemned. A drug given in these circumstances confuses the clinical picture for patient and staff alike. The effect is to commit the woman to delivery although she may not be in labour. Eventually this may involve an unnecessary caesarean section. Whosoever administers the first drug in a delivery unit assumes a grave responsibility and should be acutely conscious of the possible adverse consequences of their action.

Preparation

A woman's attitude to childbirth reflects many and varied influences to which she has been exposed since childhood. No short course of lectures is likely to result in a radical change of attitudes so deeply entrenched. Nevertheless, it would be difficult to exaggerate the importance attached to antenatal education in the alleviation of pain in labour. The general aim is to convince the expectant mother that she has nothing to fear and that she is quite capable of giving birth to her own child. This is always subject to two firm assurances: that duration of labour is limited and that personal attention is available at all times. Consciously or otherwise, these are the considerations that weigh most heavily on the mind of a woman confronted with the birth of her first child. Consequently, no effort is spared to ensure that every primigravida attends these classes on the clear understanding that the first experience of childbirth is a matter of monumental importance to the long-term happiness of the individual and her family.

Summary

The relief of pain in labour is considered under four separate headings: antenatal preparation, personal attention, limitation of duration, and analgesic drugs. The ability to restrict duration is crucial because duration of exposure to stress is the most important element in the problem of pain in labour. The duration of labour also has repercussions under each of the other three headings: antenatal preparation suffers from a serious loss of credibility when teachers are unable to state the duration of labour without the customary evasions; personal attention cannot be provided for everyone unless the commitment is limited in time; and the dosage of analgesic drugs required corresponds very closely with the hours spent in the labour ward.

16

Antenatal Preparation

Although few obstetricians nowadays appear openly hostile to the principle of preparation for childbirth, many continue to pay lip service to the ideal, while taking no interest whatsoever in the practice. This is a characteristic feature of the passive approach to management of labour, where everything will hopefully come right on the day, and should this prove not to be the case, there are few problems not amenable to treatment with analgesia—provided enough is given and by the proper route—and, failing this, there is always caesarean section. This can fittingly be described as the less-one-knows-the-better school of thought which stems from lack of direct involvement in labour management.

The almost total neglect of antenatal preparation as a legitimate topic for discussion in academic circles and the consequent lack of any authoritative guidance on organization, content or even personnel involved is indicative of the state of apathy that exists within the medical establishment regarding this important matter. Meanwhile, obstetric physiotherapists, in particular, are left very much to themselves and suffer greatly as a result, in terms of both job satisfaction for the individual and professional status for the group. Direct involvement in management, on the other hand, must lead to the conclusion that antenatal preparation is an absolutely essential element of good care in labour.

Purpose

The main purpose of antenatal preparation is and should always be seen to be to define a woman's role in labour and to teach her how to fulfil it. There are two distinct, albeit closely related components: education and training. The educational component seeks to ensure that every expectant mother has a broad understanding of the birth process, while the training component aims to teach her how to achieve the goal of spontaneous delivery.

Practice

In this hospital expectant mothers are strongly encouraged in the belief that they are well able to give birth to their own children, always provided that continuous, sympathetic and informed support is forthcoming and that

64

labour is not allowed to last too long. Thus a spirit of self-reliance is nurtured, for which these two assurances are considered necessary.

Content

The education component is based on a clear description of the first and the second stages of labour, couched in language that a lay person of reasonable intelligence can readily understand: how the one is concerned solely with the opening of the neck of the womb, a long and tedious preliminary process over which the mother has virtually no control, and the other with the passage of the infant through the birth canal, culminating in the actual birth, a short and somewhat stormy process which can be brought to a rapid conclusion by her own considerable efforts. A point to which great importance is attached is that everyone should be prepared for the sometimes cataclysmic sensation of sudden pressure on the pelvic floor which marks the transition between phase one and phase two of the second stage of labour. This is a dramatic event, which can have an altogether devastating effect when it occurs without due warning.

The concept of the graphic representation of labour is explained in some detail and mothers are shown how this is utilized to record the rate of progress and forecast the time of delivery in clinical practice. Every mother is given a copy of the partograph to take home for further study and all are expected to be familiar with the procedure when eventually admitted in labour. The simple partograph illustrated in Section II has proved an indispensable educational instrument.

The common forms of medical intervention and the reasons for them are explained: artificial rupture of membranes, oxytocin infusion, low forceps and episiotomy. A sharp distinction is made between induction of labour and treatment of abnormal uterine action after labour has already begun.

Pain is discussed briefly as a subsidiary item. To place pain in its natural context, attention is drawn to Braxton Hicks' contractions of the uterus, which are noticeable during late pregnancy, and an explanation is given as to the similarity of these with contractions of the uterus that occur during labour. The effect of anxiety on the threshold for pain is discussed. But care is taken not to make pain appear the central issue lest a serious disservice be done, which could justify the criticism that some antenatal classes are worse than none at all because women are left even more apprehensive than before. This is another aspect of the negative or passive attitude to labour.

The steps taken to supervise the condition of the child are outlined: colour of liquor and direct auscultation of heart—with scalp electrode and capillary blood sample in doubtful circumstances.

Three specific items are regarded as of such outstanding practical importance that they are covered in the form of direct questions and answers, as follows:

Question: How will you know when to go to hospital in labour?
Answer: When I get painful contractions that resemble period pains together

with a 'show' or persistent leakage of water—or, failing either of these, when the pains come at regular intervals of ten minutes or less.
Question: How long will you be there before your baby is born?
Answer: Six hours, on average, and never longer than 12 hours.
Question: Will you ever be left alone?
Answer: Never.

That every woman close to the birth of her first child should be in possession of these basic facts is considered to be the best simple test of the relevance of her preparation.

The training component is based on learning how to relax as the uterus contracts during the first stage and how to reinforce the natural expulsive forces as the uterus contracts during the second stage.

Organization

As in other areas of medical activity, careful preparation can make the difference between success and comparative failure. Attention should be concentrated on primigravidae, who form a distinct group of expectant mothers with special problems, which they approach largely with an open mind. Generally classes should be confined to primigravidae on the basis of the proposition that if one looks after the first-time mothers well, the others will look after themselves. Multigravidae should be segregated wherever possible because, as a group, their problems are quite different and alas all too often they are prejudiced by past events. Not unnaturally, a parous woman who seeks advice in this direction, especially when it is for the first time, is likely to be motivated by an unfortunate previous episode. This chain of events can have an unsettling effect on her primigravid sisters, especially when she is in the habit of recounting her own experiences, which often undermine the position of the teacher, because descriptions given in class do not correspond exactly with her memories in every minor detail. Parous women tend to have closed minds on the subject of labour. They are wont to extrapolate from what is a unique occasion in terms of personal experience and they are frequently mistaken in the belief that others placed in a similar situation would necessarily share the same point of view, even if the circumstances were identical; they do not, in a word, appreciate that women differ as much as labours. Classes for multigravidae therefore should be held separately. Indeed, a constant theme stressed throughout this manual is the need to recognize fundamental differences between primigravidae and multigravidae in everything that appertains to labour. Antenatal education must also take these differences into account.

In the case of a multigravida the main function of the teacher should be to convince her of the simple truth: that a first and a subsequent labour are not comparable in any way. This is an exercise in rehabilitation and it is well to appreciate that uncritical approval of epidural anaesthesia to solve a problem that in reality does not exist undermines a woman's self-confidence still further—no matter how grateful she may appear to be.

In this hospital, classes are arranged to correspond with antenatal clinics so that it is possible to attend both at the same visit, with the minimum of inconvenience. Attendance is limited to 24 persons and a total of 13 courses are run concurrently, both in the morning and in the afternoon, each week. Specially adapted, two of these courses are for multigravidae. The courses begin at 30 weeks so that the newfound knowledge may remain fresh in mind. Discussion is encouraged but much time is saved by anticipating the questions that are sure to be asked. Six sessions of one hour each are devoted to labour. The number of classes is restricted because as classes increase in number so do defaulters. Strict limitation on the number of classes also helps to concentrate the minds of both audience and teacher and thus to reduce the tendency to boredom. Three classes cover an understanding of the physical process of childbirth and three classes the practice of relaxation and propulsion at the appropriate times. A documentary film is shown, at which husbands are welcome, and there is a conducted tour of the delivery unit. Almost 80% of primigravidae avail themselves of this service.

Personnel

To achieve full potential, antenatal education must be conducted under enlightened medical supervision, so as to ensure that the efforts of teachers are co-ordinated and that the content is relevant to clinical practice in the institution served. This is to presuppose that clinical practice is consistent, for if it were not, it is difficult to imagine how teachers could function effectively. Teachers should be drawn from nurse-midwives and physiotherapists who have practical experience in the delivery unit in question. These disciplines correspond broadly with the educational and training components already mentioned. No teacher should be engaged exclusively in this pursuit because this would inevitably lead to a condition of isolation, which is one of the main factors militating against proper recognition of antenatal educational services in general.

As mutual trust is the keynote, this requires that teachers appear not only to know precisely what they are talking about in strictly medical terms and in relation to practice in the particular institution, but also to have insight into the anxieties peculiar to a group of women faced with the challenge of a lifetime. Furthermore, teachers should be acutely conscious of the exceptional opportunity afforded to them to provide a favourable image of the overall service to the consumer. All too often teachers and practitioners appear to be in conflict with each other because they have little or no common ground.

Summary

Antenatal classes have now been available on an organized basis for a considerable time without meeting with the level of acceptance that they so obviously deserve. There are genuine reasons for this comparative failure that need to be carefully examined, with a view to placing the service on a more acceptable footing all round. This development would be of enormous benefit to everyone concerned with the conduct of labour. The ambivalent nature of medical opinion seems to derive mainly from the conviction that much of what is taught is irrelevant if not downright harmful, while this is met by the countercharge that there is very little in the form of consistent medical practice to be relevant to in most institutions. Worst of all is the frequency with which two indispensable arms of the same service appear to operate at loggerheads.

17

Analgesic Drugs

Pethidine is the standard drug for the relief of pain in labour and is used almost everywhere. Although far from ideal for the purpose, it has been tested on such an extensive scale that it is generally agreed to be about the best drug available and comparatively safe in reasonable doses. Safety is of paramount importance, particularly as it relates to the child, and this should preclude the use of new preparations until exhaustive clinical trials have been performed. It is notable that despite numerous initial claims to the contrary, no drug has yet emerged to challenge the dominant position of pethidine. The reason for this is that the ability of a drug to relieve pain is directly proportional to its adverse effects, especially on the respiratory centre of the newborn. Pethidine is the only drug used to relieve pain in labour in this hospital.

Disadvantages of Pethidine

Pethidine has many disadvantages and these are wholly unpredictable in individual cases. Some women suffer from intractable nausea and vomiting sufficient to turn childbirth into a miserable experience. Some become profoundly depressed, introspective and so overwhelmed with self-pity that they lapse into a state of semiconsciousness, from which they are roused only by contractions to make aimless protests and demand more and more drugs, until the original situation is compounded and a vicious circle is established. Some become completely disorientated and so confused that they are quite unable to co-operate with their attendants, particularly during the second stage of labour, when co-operation is essential if spontaneous delivery is to be achieved. Spontaneous delivery represents an important personal achievement, of which mothers should not lightly be deprived, and it also provides the best possible insurance against trauma.

In practice, many women in labour are deeply intoxicated; out of bed they would be unable to stand upright and would certainly be deemed unfit to drive a car. Like drunken persons everywhere, they are likely to suffer from a hangover, which is a most undesirable sequel to such a joyous occasion as a birth especially of a first child. All these unpleasant effects may follow even a small dose of pethidine in a person who has had no previous experience of hard drugs. Unfortunately, the unpleasant effects of pethidine have become closely identified with labour in the popular mind. Paradoxically, this leads to an even greater demand for drugs.

The most serious effect of pethidine is on the child. Depression of the respiratory centre may delay the establishment of normal breathing in the critical minutes after birth. This can result in brain damage, especially in preterm infants and where adequate facilities for resuscitation are not available at all times. Sophisticated methods of examination reveal subtle changes in behaviour in the newborn after what most obstetricians would regard as homeopathic doses of pethidine. These changes raise the question as to whether pethidine, however small the dose, is entirely safe for the child.

A question that needs to be asked is whether the advantages of pethidine are outweighed by its disadvantages to the extent that its use in labour should be discontinued completely. The plain fact of the matter, however, is that it is simply not possible to provide sufficient pethidine to relieve pain in labour effectively without introducing an extraneous element of discomfort and sometimes danger. The problem is that there is no more suitable drug available. The treatment of pain in labour must therefore of necessity entail a genuine compromise between a reasonable degree of analgesia and a reasonable element of extraneous discomfort in the mother, with depression of the nervous system in the infant.

A number of drugs have been recommended in combination with pethidine in the hope that they might enhance the desirable or neutralize the undesirable effects. None has proved successful. As a matter of medical principle, drugs in combination are best avoided because they cross the placenta, confuse the diagnosis of fetal distress, and cause serious problems in the newborn, which can last for a considerable time: diazepam, which can be detected weeks later, is a good recent example.

Naloxone is a specific opiate antagonist which competes at receptor level and therefore reverses all the effects of pethidine, including the desired analgesic effect, within minutes of injection. Consequently its application during labour is limited, but it can be invaluable after delivery, particularly in the case of the newborn, in reversing pethidine-induced respiratory depression. Its only drawback appears to be a short half-life, which could require that it be infused over a period of time.

Use of Pethidine

Pethidine should not be used on a routine basis simply to comply with an obstetric ritual or to protect staff from possible criticism later. A doctor who seems critical of a nurse-midwife because an occasional woman subsequently complains that she has not had sufficient relief from pain encourages this form of mass medication. Doctors are seldom present to witness the circumstances and it is all too easy for them to pose as more humane after the event. No personal commitment is required for this. The strongest arguments in favour of large doses of analgesic drugs in labour are usually advanced by doctors who do not themselves spend much time in a delivery unit. Pethidine, it must be emphasized, often makes labour more unpleasant than it otherwise would have been, and the more pethidine a woman receives, the more disgruntled she often becomes. Indeed, the woman who complains most vehemently is not infrequently the victim of a surfeit of drugs.

The practice in this hospital is to await the reaction of each woman to her own experience of labour. Everyone is treated as an individual in this respect. Expectant mothers are advised that all methods of pain relief are available, but that prior commitments are not given because they are considered not to serve the best interests of the individual. Expectant mothers are, however, given a firm assurance that the duration of labour will be strictly limited and that a personal nurse will be present at all times: they are, in other words, encouraged to consider the problem of pain relief in a much wider context. In practice, the result is that one-half of all primigravidae and many more multigravidae request no analgesic drugs whatsoever during labour.

First Stage

Pethidine is given only with the informed consent of the mother and then during the first stage of labour. The initial dose is 50 mg. This serves as a test dose to assess the individual's response. A small dose is preferred because should a larger dose be given and side-effects caused, the error cannot easily be rectified. Adequate relief for the duration of the first stage of labour is provided by a single injection of 50 mg in a high proportion of cases. A second injection is given half an hour later if the effect is not adequate and side-effects are not troublesome. The total dose of pethidine never exceeds 100 mg, and whenever this proves inadequate an epidural block is introduced. Pethidine in excess of 100 mg, tends to cause more discomfort than it relieves. No alternative drug is used and no combination of drugs is permitted. This exercise of strict control over the distribution of analgesic drugs fosters a much more constructive approach to the whole wearisome problem of stress in labour.

Second Stage

There is not nearly the same need for analgesia during the second stage of labour because during contractions mothers are generally preoccupied with the task in hand. This distraction operates as a most effective method of pain relief. The sense of frustration so typical of the first stage is now replaced by a burst of activity, through which a woman can largely determine her own fate. Properly harnessed, this awareness can alter her whole outlook. There are two exceptions to this general observation: (i) during phase one of the second stage, before the baby's head has descended to the level at which the push reflex is activated, when nothing extra in the way of drugs is required because this is merely an extension of the first stage of labour; and (ii) late in phase two, as the head crowns, when there is clearly a need for something more.

The drug used in this hospital for the relief of pain during phase two of the second stage of labour was until recently trilene. Trilene was preferred to nitrous oxide because, while equally effective and safe, it had the additional advantages of being both portable and cheap. Like nitrous oxide, it was dispensed by the patient herself, who regulated the dose by the depth of her breathing and by the tightness with which the mask was held to her face. As the manufacture of trilene was about to be discontinued, there seemed to be no option but to change to nitrous oxide, which is neither portable nor cheap. Meanwhile, trilene continues to be produced. But whatever the drug, inhalation analgesia is confined strictly to phase two and is used only for a short period of time lest longer exposure should lead to hyperventilation with alkalosis and dehydration, and a severe hangover effect. The benefit of inhalation analgesia is most apparent as the baby's head crowns, although even then it often appears to act more as a source of distraction and an inducement to breathe rather than push at this critical juncture.

Forceps delivery is always conducted under pudendal block, for two main reasons: first, because the not inconsiderable risk of a general anaesthetic given to a woman advanced in labour is eliminated, and second, because strict limitation is automatically placed on the scope for manoeuvre by the operator, with a consequent reduction in the likelihood of trauma. There is, in addition, the practical advantage of not requiring the presence of an anaesthetist. Rotation with forceps is not permitted and for this reason Kielland's forceps are not available in this hospital.

Summary

The ideal drug for the relief of pain in labour does not exist. Pethidine is the best available. But it is open to serious question whether pethidine may not cause more discomfort than it relieves. A far more critical approach to the whole question of drugs in labour is desirable. Certainly no drug whatsoever should be given until a firm diagnosis of labour has been made and the woman is therefore committed to delivery. Pain should not be considered as a separate problem in total isolation from other very relevant aspects of labour. Alternative methods of relief—notably antenatal preparation, continuous personal attention and strict control of duration—offer much brighter prospects for future development.

18

Epidural Anaesthesia

Epidural anaesthesia, as the term implies, affords complete relief of pain in all but a few instances and has the decided additional advantage that it is not associated with any of the unpleasant side-effects of pethidine. The mother retains her mental acuity and the infant is alert at birth. There are few more impressive sights than the resolution of maternal stress that follows a successful epidural block in labour. The answer to the problem of maternal stress in labour might therefore appear simple: make epidural anaesthesia available on a universal basis and encourage everyone to avail themselves of the service. However, this would be gross over-simplification of a much more complex problem, because although epidural block is far more effective than pethidine, it is also far more dangerous. No good purpose is served by pretending otherwise. The dangers of epidural anaesthesia can be considered under two headings: direct effects of a local anaesthetic solution placed in the epidural space; and indirect effects of the anaesthesia on the course of labour.

Direct Adverse Effects

The main danger of epidural block is accidental entry of the anaesthetic solution into the cerebrospinal fluid. This can lead to profound depression of vital centres, collapse of circulation and even death. There is also the possibility of permanent damage among survivors. The likelihood of a disaster of such magnitude largely depends on the skill and experience of the anaesthetist, but it cannot be entirely excluded, because the mechanism is inherent in the procedure itself. The risk of any form of medical intervention in current obstetric practice must be measured against the background of one maternal death for every 10 000 babies born. Two deaths in a series of 10 000 mothers who received an epidural block would represent an increase of 100% in the maternal mortality rate in developed countries. No series of this magnitude has been published, and if it were, it would still be less than adequate from a statistical viewpoint. Published series, moreover, are almost always presented by specialist anaesthetists, operating under ideal conditions in teaching hospitals. Furthermore, they are concerned only with the direct effects of the procedure that fall within their own area of competence. Even so, there is a notable reluctance to publish details of maternal catastrophes that occur in association with epidural anaesthesia and an understandable tendency to attribute these to intercurrent disease such as toxaemia, haemorrhage and ruptured uterus, where possible without sufficient regard to the fact that epidural block can play a critical role in the response of the organism to these conditions. There is a grey area between anaesthetics and obstetrics into which not a few disasters of childbirth fall. Severe headache following dural tap and retention of urine requiring repeated catheterization are less serious but nevertheless disturbing consequences encountered more frequently than is generally appreciated in postnatal wards, thus casting a cloud over a period of otherwise greatest joy.

Indirect Adverse Effects

The obstetrician must also be concerned with the indirect effects of epidural anaesthesia on the course of labour. This is an aspect of the procedure to which far too little attention is paid.

Sometimes epidural anaesthesia is given too early, before a firm diagnosis of labour has been made. The result is that, after much confusion, a caesarean section is eventually performed on a woman who is not in labour, because it is wellnigh impossible to withdraw an epidural anaesthetic before delivery. Usually the mistake is not recognized, but even so the obstetrician would be understandably slow to admit that a woman has had an unnecessary caesarean section to retrieve a situation caused by a palliative procedure, the implications of which she may not have fully understood. Although the operation is performed to retrieve an iatrogenic situation, the need for caesarean section is attributed to lack of progress in labour. The effect of this is to transfer the onus to the patient. Hence an epidural anaesthetic should never be given until a firm diagnosis of labour has been made and the woman is therefore committed to delivery. This should effectively preclude epidural anaesthesia before an attempt is made to induce labour.

Sometimes epidural anaesthesia is given too late, when the cervix is near full dilatation. The result is that the beneficial effects in the first stage of labour are more than offset by the adverse effects in the second stage. The benefits of epidural block are reaped almost entirely during the first stage and the price is paid largely during the second stage. This price is manifest in the form of a sharp increase in the number of forceps deliveries, with the associated risk of trauma. The problem of the late epidural is more likely to arise in the case of a parous woman to whom a prior commitment has been made and who in the event expects that the commitment be honoured, come what may. This is especially likely when an element of subtle persuasion has been involved to influence the woman to the viewpoint that to make childbirth a tolerable experience epidural anaesthesia is necessary.

Sometimes epidural anaesthesia is used as a palliative procedure when labour is prolonged, as if duration itself were not important provided that the mother suffers no pain. This approach to the subject of pain illustrates the fundamental difference between the philosophies that underlie active and passive management of labour. The active management of labour is based on the proposition that the risks increase as the duration of labour increases, whether or not a woman suffers pain. The total relief of pain can create a false sense of security when labour is prolonged. Rupture of the uterus is the ultimate expression of trauma in the mother and epidural anaesthesia has emerged as an important factor in the aetiology of this calamity in recent years. Rupture of the uterus is virtually confined to multigravidae and it is very significant that the first reported case of rupture of the uterus attributed to oxytocin in a primigravida occurred under cover of epidural anaesthesia after 54 hours in labour, as described in Chapter 14. This was a classic example of the misuse of epidural to permit the duration of labour to be extended for a dangerous length of time. Ironically, the declared purpose of the publication of the details of the case in the medical literature was to prove the contrary to what is asserted here: that it is indeed possible to rupture a primigravid uterus with oxytocin. The firm recommendation is that epidural anaesthesia should not be used as a substitute for corrective action in prolonged labour.

Epidural anaesthesia results in a sharp increase in the number of forceps deliveries. Some 10% of primigravidae are delivered with forceps in this hospital, compared with as many as 70% in centres where epidural anaesthesia is freely used. Traumatic intracranial haemorrhage is the ultimate expression of trauma in the child. Apart from breech presentation, this is associated almost invariabably with forceps application. The risk of trauma is greatest when the baby's head is transverse and rotation is effected. But it cannot be overemphasized that trauma in cephalic presentation is inflicted with instruments and that it is not a problem in spontaneous delivery. Epidural anaesthesia therefore has an important bearing on trauma to the child because it greatly reduces the likelihood of spontaneous delivery.

The number of spontaneous deliveries can be increased when there is the will to do so. Motivation to this end largely depends on a clear appreciation of the importance of mothers giving birth to their own children. The incidence of forceps deliveries, however, is unlikely to be reduced much below 50% in primigravidae who have received epidural anaesthesia. The magnitude of the increase is likely to be overlooked if the figure is diluted by the addition of multigravidae, who rarely require forceps delivery in any event.

The inevitable loss of mobility associated with epidural block can be a considerable disadvantage.

Case Selection

In some centres epidural anaesthesia is not given to those who may require it simply because it is not always available, while in other centres it is given to those who do not require it simply because it is there. Once what has become known as an epidural service has been established and additional personnel employed, there are hidden pressures to increase the number of cases merely to justify the existence of the service. Epidural block is available at all times in this hospital as an integral part of the service, but availability is not a factor that determines its use. A genuine attempt was made to define a role for epidural anaesthesia, and while no claims to scientific accuracy are made, because any such study is of necessity based on mainly subjective criteria, the conclusions reached nevertheless provide a better working guide for patients and staff than the whims of either of the parties that so often determine practice in this sphere.

The first conclusion was that epidural anaesthesia has an invaluable contribution to make to the management of labour in some primigravidae, but, equally important, that it has no contribution to make to the management of labour in multigravidae. The use of epidural anaesthesia in multigravidae stems from the mistaken belief that any valid comparison can be drawn between a first and a subsequent labour. A woman who has had an unpleasant first experience of labour, during which she may or may not have had an epidural anaesthetic, frequently seeks a prior commitment on the next occasion because she fears that the experience is likely to be repeated. There are no grounds whatsoever for such misapprehension. The obstetrician would serve the interests of the parous woman much better were he to allay her fears with a simple explanation of the essential difference between a first and a subsequent birth. This course would also save his anaesthetist colleague from the embarrassment of having his efforts to retrieve the prior commitment entered into by the obstetrician interrupted by the untimely arrival of the infant, often at dead of night. Moreover, it is in parous women that epidural anaesthesia acts to increase the risk of a ruptured uterus, partly because the parous uterus is prone and partly because pain has an important protective function in this regard. These are compelling reasons why epidural anaesthesia should be confined to primigravidae.

The second conclusion was that it is most unwise to enter into a prior commitment, even with a primigravida, because this constitutes a tacit encouragement to a negative or passive attitude to labour. Prior commitment becomes especially undesirable when it is adopted as a policy to be propagated through antenatal educational channels. There are two sound reasons why an expectant approach to epidural anaesthesia should be practised: first, the reaction of each individual to the actual experience of a first labour can rarely be foretold, perhaps least of all by herself; and second, the duration of labour cannot be predicted. Some 40% of primigravidae are delivered within four hours of admission to this hospital without treatment of any sort. And included in this time is the second stage of labour, when the effects of epidural block are almost wholly adverse. The second stage is tolerated much better than the first because mothers can exercise a more assertive role. Besides, there are not many women who genuinely wish to be deprived of the sense of achievement that comes from giving birth to their first child.

Subject to these two strong reservations—that epidural block be confined to primigravidae and that prior commitments not be given—the women who derived most benefit from epidural anaesthesia fell into three more or less distinct groups, as follows: (i) those who were so disturbed at the very prospect of labour that they were already unduly upset at the point of admission; (ii) those who, despite initial composure, became unduly upset soon afterwards; and (iii) those who were not in sight of delivery after six hours. The number in the first group was closely related to antenatal preparation, the number in the second group to the quality of care after admission, and the number in the third group to the duration of labour. Approximately 5% of primigravidae were included in one or other of these three groups, and the incidence of epidural anaesthesia in this hospital has remained remarkably constant at this level for several years past.

With one exception, epidural block is used only for the relief of pain. The exception is the case of a woman with an uncontrollable desire to push against a cervix that has not reached full dilatation. Epidural block is not used as a form of therapy in systemic diseases, such as chronic hypertension or pre-eclampsia, or in obstetric abnormalities, such as breech presentation or twins.

Responsibility

The question of ultimate responsibility for epidural block deserves more serious consideration than it has yet received, especially where a prior commitment has been given and where the person involved is a parous woman. Can it be presumed that the mother, in requesting an epidural anaesthetic, gives blanket acceptance to all the consequences, direct and indirect, without being in a position to fully understand and therefore, it can reasonably be said, without being fully informed? And how far does the obstetrician meet his professional obligation by sanctioning the procedure several months in advance and therefore without due regard to the particular circumstances at the time of administration? And what of the anaesthetist summoned to provide an emergency service, with little or no knowledge of the background, obstetric or otherwise? Finally, and because timing is so critical, there is the nurse-midwife, whose decision may be of vital importance, particularly in the case of a parous woman. These are issues that do not arise when the decision to use epidural anaesthesia is made on a selective basis during the course of labour.

Summary

Epidural block has a special contribution to make to the management of labour in a select number of cases. It should, however, be regarded as an exceptional measure and treated always with due respect. The risks are not confined to the technical procedure itself but also encompass the patient's ability to respond to shock. The greatly increased need for assisted delivery has a major impact on obstetric practice. There is the real possibility of rupture of the uterus in multigravidae. Epidural block should therefore be restricted to primigravidae, given not too early or too late, and not used as a cover for prolonged labour. Consequently, not more than two doses should be needed. Prior commitments should not be given. With one exception, epidural block should not be used as a therapeutic agent, but only for the relief of pain.

19
Personal Attention

One of the most disturbing prospects of labour is fear of isolation, which the mere mention of a delivery unit seems to engender in many women. This fear is certainly not a reflection on the standard of medical practice as ordinarily understood, rather the problem tends to increase as technical standards rise. The more efficient a hospital in strictly medical terms, the more isolated the mothers are likely to feel. The result is that the general public seems to have reached the conclusion that medical efficiency and humane considerations are not compatible. Nowadays in obstetrics, to be called efficient has to be regarded as a doubtful compliment.

Moral Support

Childbirth is a unique event that should provide a sense of profound and lasting satisfaction for mothers, in which nurse-midwives and doctors can share. Yet, as it happens, there are many mothers who complain bitterly of the apparent indifference of the very ones in whom they placed their trust during the most vulnerable hours of their lives. Those closest to the action often do not appear to realize that there are few places on earth so lonely as a busy delivery unit. The human consciousness is seldom more open to impression than during the long hours of labour, and a casual approach to just another routine assignment may leave a mother with a burning sense of resentment. Apparently trivial events like a curt tone of voice, a bloodstained glove, mindless exposure in the indelicate lithotomy position or failure to convey the result of a pelvic examination directly, though not of great consequence in themselves, portray an often deplorable lack of sensitivity in professional staff who should know much better. Because of a heightened sense of awareness at this time, the memory of these affronts to personal dignity, unintentional though they may be, are none the less preserved indefinitely and in photographic detail by many women.

The steady emotional decline which is a characteristic feature of labour not properly supervised follows an entirely predictable course. The scenario can be written in advance. The woman becomes progressively withdrawn from contact with her surroundings, closes her eyes and buries her face in the pillow, only later to become increasingly active, with contorted features and restless movements interrupted by frantic outbursts, until finally a state of panic is reached and self-control is lost completely. Once the morale of a woman in labour has begun to crumble it becomes more and more difficult to restore the balance. Nurses, in particular, must always be conscious of the need to keep every woman in labour on a tight emotional rein from the time of her admission until the baby is born, because the further she is allowed to slip down the emotional incline the more difficult it is for her to recover composure. Specifically, women in labour must be encouraged to keep their eyes open at all times, because closed eyes usually mark the first step on the road to total disintegration. The best protection possible against the gradual erosion of a woman's personal dignity in labour is to hold her attention firmly the outset.

Panic, which may sometimes be suppressed only by a general anaesthetic, is a shattering experience from which a person may never fully recover. This may lead to recurrent nightmares, permanent revulsion to childbirth, with consequent marital disharmony, and a sense of antagonism even towards her own child. Not nearly enough attention has been paid to this aspect of trauma in childbirth. It should be considered as one of the most serious complications in obstetrics—more serious than a ruptured uterus in many ways—and should never be allowed to happen. Much less serious emotional trauma than this has caused some misguided women to advocate a return to home confinement, while freely acknowledging that the purely medical case in favour of hospital confinement is overwhelming. Consequently, there is an urgent need to recognize that a profound fear of isolation during labour is widespread, to acknowledge that the fear is only too well founded in practice, and to resolve that something effective must be done to rectify this unfortunate situation.

The Nurse-Midwife

The only solution to the dread of isolation is a prior guarantee to every expectant mother of continuous personal attention through labour.

Personal attention in this sense means one nurse to one patient, face to face. What personal attention does not mean is a group of nurses caring for a equal number of patients on a collective basis. Although the total number of nurses deployed in a delivery unit may be more than adequate on paper, many women still complain of being left alone for comparatively long periods of time. Positive steps are therefore necessary to ensure that each woman in labour identifies by name with an individual nurse. Although the physical presence of a trained companion is in itself a source of considerable comfort to the woman in labour, mere physical presence is not nearly enough. The nurse must appreciate that her primary duty to the mother is to provide the emotional support so badly needed at this critical time and not simply to record vital signs in a detached clinical manner. The physical condition of the mother must of course be supervised. But this is simply a matter of recording vital signs at regular intervals of two hours. These particular records have very little relevance to the great majority of healthy women, who are delivered within hours of admission. In many centres an altogether disproportionate amount of space on the partograph is allotted to such observations, seemingly to make provision for the possibility that every woman in labour might suffer from eclampsia.

The real value of a personal nurse is best reflected in the facial expression of a woman in labour. Each nurse must consciously strive to establish a strong sense of rapport with her patient by seeking to identify topics of common interest. By far the most impressive evidence of the quality of care afforded in a delivery unit is to watch nurse and mother engage in animated conversation and exchange smiles in the process. Smiles are more effective than drugs in the relief of pain in labour. Some individuals are obviously better than others in the field of human relationships, but almost everyone can become proficient when they are sufficiently aware of the need. A woman's experience of labour depends to a very great extent on the personal relationship established with her nurse. The nurse on the other hand derives her greatest satisfaction from the opportunity to contribute so much to someone under duress. Those who share moments of stress tend to forge a lasting bond and it is truly remarkable how often a woman can recall the kindness of a particular nurse many years after her first confinement. Naturally communication is much easier in the context of a common culture. Although likely to be more difficult when the cultural background of the nurse differs widely from that of her patient, failure to communicate in any real sense of the word arises much more often from the nurse not having been trained to appreciate the need. Specifically, every nurse has a responsibility to ensure that her patient genuinely understands the purpose of every medical procedure and the result of every examination, and that she is kept informed of progress, with regular updating of the time at which her baby is expected to be born.

A guarantee is given to every expectant mother who attends this hospital that she will have a personal nurse through the whole of labour, from the time of her admission until after her baby is born, without regard to the hour of day or night. Many mothers, and observers too, believe this to be the most important development in management of labour in recent years. But they do not always realize that it would not be feasible unless the duration of labour were limited. The authors rate personal attention as second only in significance to the limitation of duration in management of labour, although the two are inseparable because one cannot be achieved without the other. With 8000 deliveries per annum, a personal nurse for every woman in labour is no mean achievement.

The Doctor

Doctors too must recognize that they also have an indispensable role to play in the provision of personal care and attention, which is a central issue in management of labour. The consultant obstetrician, who is ultimately responsible for the overall welfare of women in labour, must set the example, because inevitably his attitude pervades the entire system. Young doctors and nurses follow the example set by their teachers. Unfortunately, on the attainment of consultant rank many obstetricians virtually abandon the delivery unit for the antenatal ward or operating theatre, and henceforth in so far as labour is concerned their attention is confined to a small number of abnormal cases of purely medical interest. Even senior residents are seldom seen in some delivery units until the need for surgical intervention arises. The result is that management of labour in normal women, who represent a large majority in any given unit, is left to junior residents, who have far less experience than senior nurses. There is absolutely no point in the consultant obstetrician advocating a standard of personal care and attention to which he is not prepared to contribute in a positive way. He must be seen to practise what he preaches. This means that he must be seen in the delivery unit at regular intervals every day and must converse directly with each woman on the questions that he should know are uppermost in her mind at this time. In other words, he must underwrite the whole ethos of labour management by personal example.

The Husband

The extent to which husbands should be encouraged to remain with their wives through the course of labour and delivery remains very much an open question. Sometimes it is difficult to avoid the impression that husbands are enlisted to protect their wives against the very fear of isolation that is the subject of the present chapter, or even to protect them from unwarranted intervention. Experience in this hospital suggests that women have much more to gain from the presence of a female companion who is not just sympathetic but well informed and therefore in a much better position to provide the firm reassurance that is so sorely needed.

Summary

A personal nurse for every woman in labour has proved itself to be a practical proposition in the busiest maternity unit in the British Isles for more than a decade past. Mothers tend to regard this as the most important single advance in the conduct of labour in recent years. Strict limitation of the duration of labour and continuous personal attention throughout are considered to be the basic requirements on which a high standard of care depends. There is a close correlation between the two, as neither is possible without the other.

20

Role of the Doctor

The role of the doctor in the management of labour needs to be considered at four quite different levels of responsibility.

Consultant Obstetricians

Consultant obstetricians are in a unique position to influence the standard of care in labour for the better, simply by agreeing on a common policy of management within the confines of each hospital. The main obstacle to improvement in the quality of care in labour in most institutions is a lack of clear direction from the top. Nurses and resident doctors are frequently placed in the invidious position of having to apply different methods of treatment in exactly the same clinical circumstances for no reason other than that the names of the consultants entered on the charts are different. A good illustration of this is when patients in adjacent beds receive different concentrations of oxytocin or different analgesic drugs for no more convincing reason than that they happen to have attended the antenatal clinic on different days. The sheer irrationality of this mode of action is a constant affront to the intelligence of professional staff. No one would dare suggest that an intensive care unit in a general hospital could operate efficiently under direction of such a capricious nature. Hence, wherever a genuine wish to improve the quality of care offered to women in labour exists, the first essential step is for the consultant obstetricians to come together and agree to surrender a small portion of their jealously guarded independence for the common good. This, the authors suggest, is the acid test of goodwill at consultant level. Without this co-operation, a delivery unit cannot even begin to achieve its full potential. Naturally, someone must take the initial step.

First in order of priority, the chain of command must be sharply defined. There should be one person only in charge of a delivery unit at any one time. A delivery unit cannot operate efficiently under the committee system. For practical reasons the person responsible must be a nurse-midwife. She should be designated as sister-in-charge and wear a distinctive uniform that can be recognized immediately by all concerned. Everyone who works in the unit should be subject to her immediate authority. There is no more room for divided responsibility in a delivery unit than there is aboard a ship at sea.

Next, the most sensitive areas of management must be clearly identified and the general outline of procedure standardized. These subjects have been addressed in previous chapters under the appropriate headings: Diagnosis, Progress, Duration, Acceleration, etc.

82

After the critical decision to delegate authority, the most valuable contribution the consultants can make to the conduct of labour is to declare full acceptance of responsibility for the outcome. There is no place for equivocation on this issue because delegation of authority on any other terms is meaningless. A bland declaration to the effect is worthless unless the individuals concerned are truly convinced that a scapegoat will not be sought whenever a mishap occurs, as sooner or later it undoubtedly will, as long as human beings remain fallible. Unfortunately this is only too often the case. And when trust is lacking decisions are avoided, treatment is not pursued effectively and caesarean sections are performed unnecessarily, because surgery provides a soft option for those anxious to avoid blame. Contrary often to superficial appearances, the decision to submit a woman to caesarean section is usually taken by resident staff before the consultant who may eventually perform the operation is even notified.

The consultant obstetrician should be at pains to show equal concern for all women in labour and not concentrate attention on the few who are abnormal. He should be conscious of the potential to boost morale by frequent appearances in the delivery unit. Meanwhile, he should not interfere in routine management, but rather encourage the nursing staff to get on with the job themselves.

Albeit facilitated greatly by the Mastership system, wherein one obstetrician is appointed to act as chief executive for a statutory period of seven years, a high level of co-operation between all ten members of the consultant staff is a well-established feature of this hospital.

Senior Residents

Senior residents hold a specialist qualification in obstetrics and gynaecology: they are four in number and there is a strict rule that one must be on the premises at all times. The most important function of the senior resident on duty in this hospital is to review the condition of every woman in labour at regular intervals of approximately four hours, particularly late at night. The senior resident is expected to be familiar with everyone in labour and not, as so often happens elsewhere, remain aloof until summoned to undertake an operative delivery. All but a few obstetric cases are normal at the point of admission, but many more subsequently become abnormal simply because they are not supervised adequately from the beginning. Most complications of labour develop in hospital and could readily have been avoided had proper care and attention been given from the time of admission. The duty of the senior resident is to ensure that this simple proposition is put into everyday practice. A good personal relationship with the sister-in-charge is an essential prerequisite to this end.

The senior resident decides, always in consultation with the sister-in-charge, when to terminate labour, and he also chooses the method of delivery, except caesarean section, which must be referred to a consultant. The need to intervene on the conventional grounds of failure to advance or maternal distress declines sharply when a policy of active management is pursued from the outset. The only two operative methods of delivery now permitted in this hospital are caesarean section and low forceps extraction, and the incidence of both procedures is unusually low by comparison with other centres. There is no longer an opportunity for trainee specialists to acquire what some would still regard as essential skills, such as forceps rotation and ventouse extraction, because these are no longer practised. Nowadays, senior residents are cast firmly in the role of obstetric physicians rather than obstetric surgeons, with most emphasis on the conduct of labour in normal women.

Junior Residents

Junior residents are in training either as specialists or as family practitioners. No junior resident is directly involved in the decision-making process in this hospital. Junior residents are cast in the role of postgraduate students, whose main function is to learn about normal birth and certainly not to teach others how to solve complicated clinical problems of which they have little experience. Most young doctors are only too relieved when this situation is frankly stated, because no intelligent young man or woman wishes to be placed in a false position, where it is necessary to adopt a pretence at expertise that he and everyone else knows he does not possess. Those who do not readily accept this situation represent a potential danger. Although a junior resident is present in the delivery unit of this hospital at all times— one of the practical advantages of scale—this is not considered a necessary feature of good management and the arrangement could be said to operate more to the advantage of the doctor himself. Junior residents are subject to the authority of the sister-in-charge and function under her supervision. The practical tasks they perform are artificial rupture of membranes, low forceps delivery and perineal repair. The sister-in-charge consults directly with the senior resident whenever she is in doubt about the management of a particular case. The junior resident is not in a position to dictate to the sister nor to overrule her decision in any matter.

Medical Students

Clinical obstetrics is presented to undergraduates in a manner that is quite different from that of former years. Nowadays the aim is purely educational. Teaching is based on the assumption that all births take place in hospital and that comparatively few doctors will ever again attend a woman in labour. Nevertheless, it is considered to be one of the fundamental requirements of medical education in the broadest sense that every doctor, no matter what discipline he may pursue in later life, should observe at close quarters the nature of childbirth and understand the implications of current management. With this in mind, every student in this medical school must work eight hours for seven consecutive days in the delivery unit, where he must provide personal care for one mother each day in a face-to-face relationship. Each medical student must function alone and one only is permitted in the delivery unit at any one time. Medical students are subject to the same discipline as student nurses. A medical student is not permitted to leave a woman in labour without the express permission of the sister-in-charge and then only when a replacement is immediately available. At the end of seven days the medical student must submit a report on every case supervised, devoting special attention to the emotional impact on the mother.

A medical student may not leave a woman in labour to observe a forceps or breech delivery, even when it is conducted in the adjoining room. He is given to understand that the commitment to a woman in labour must be absolute and that it is the very negation of good teaching to make use of a woman in labour for one's own advantage, only to abandon her when something more spectacular comes along. This is usually the first and probably the only occasion in the whole medical curriculum when a student comes face to face with a person under severe emotional stress for a protracted period of time and almost all agree that it is a salutary experience that can be turned to good effect in other branches of medicine. Medical students are immensely gratified to find how much can be achieved by personal commitment in this field. This close encounter with individuals under stress is regarded as the essence of undergraduate teaching on the subject of labour. No longer are medical students exposed to the obstetrical curiosities and the complicated deliveries. The emphasis is on normal labour and it is seen as no function of undergraduate teaching to produce a doctor qualified to commence practice in obstetrics on the day of graduation. A future family practitioner who may wish to provide antenatal and postnatal care in conjunction with a hospital is required to serve at least six months as a junior resident.

Summary

Consultant obstetricians who cannot agree on a common overall policy of management represent possibly the main impediment to improved standards of care in labour at the present time. The purpose of this manual is to outline such an overall policy and to show how it was put into practice in one large teaching centre. To be successful it is absolutely essential that the role of the junior resident be re-defined as that of a postgraduate student, and that, as such, he be integrated into the team at an appropriate level. The attention of undergraduates needs to be directed more to the emotional impact of labour and less to the occasional technical manoeuvres, which are devoid of all educational value.

21

Role of the Nurse-Midwife

The role of the nurse in the management of labour is considered at three levels in this hospital. A sister-in-charge and a staff nurse-midwife are both state registered general nurses and trained midwives at different levels of experience. A pupil nurse-midwife is also a state registered nurse, having completed three years in an accredited general hospital and passed a public examination. Midwifery is a postgraduate subject, which requires two additional years practical experience and a similar examination. There are 100 pupil midwives in this hospital at any time, an intake of 50 per annum. This number constitutes approximately one-half of the entire nursing staff. Wherever the terms 'nurse' and 'midwife' are used in this text they should be regarded as interchangeable, because all are general trained and either trained or trainee midwives.

Sister-in-Charge

The sister-in-charge of the delivery unit is of paramount importance and it is openly acknowledged that hers is a vital role. In practice, she must make all the critical decisions in management, which otherwise would not be made. She must confirm or reject the diagnosis of labour in every case admitted. She must measure dilatation of the cervix at regular intervals. She must decide when to accelerate slow progress. And she must carry these decisions into effect—day and night—without reference to medical staff who may be otherwise engaged, when not asleep in bed. Finally, she must decide when the limits of her authority have been reached and seek consultation. All this adds up to a formidable responsibility, which requires strength of character as well as years of experience.

When the sister-in-charge decides that the limits of her authority have been reached, the opportunity for consultation with a medical colleague of comparable status is readily available. It would be utterly incongruous if a nurse with such wide experience of a very specialized nature were placed in the position of having to seek the advice of a junior resident, who holds a primary medical qualification. The practical experience of the average junior resident is restricted to hasty appearances at normal births during a short period of undergraduate residence, possibly instructed by the selfsame nurse.

The sister-in-charge of this delivery unit is vested with the authority necessary to perform the duties of her office effectively. Specifically, she does not consult with any doctor below the status of senior resident. As each sister-in-charge is personally responsible for some 1500 deliveries per annum, she is recognized as an expert in the field and her advice is keenly sought by members of the medical staff on all aspects of labour.

The influence of the sister-in-charge is no less important at a humane level. The air of quiet efficiency that is the hallmark of a good delivery unit depends on her. This intangible element, which communicates itself so easily to others, is an essential ingredient of the spirit of mutual trust that is such a necessary component of good management. Mothers need to sense that nurses and doctors, to whose care they are committed during these difficult hours, behave as members of a team, each with a known part to play. As captain of the team, no one compares in importance with the sister-in-charge, so she surely has the right to expect the unqualified support of her colleagues—doctors as well as nurses—in this onerous task. A delivery unit cannot begin to function smoothly without a strong team spirit and everyone suffers when this is lacking.

In addition to one overall supervisor, there are five nurses with the rank of sister-in-charge of the delivery unit employed in this hospital. There is always one on duty, day and night, and only one to guard against the possible adverse effects of a division of responsibility. The result is that each sister-in-charge works for on average one-fifth part of each week: the equivalent of 33 hours and 36 minutes. The actual hours worked are flexible and are left largely to the discretion of those directly involved. There is no permanent night duty. The sister-in-charge of the delivery unit devotes her undivided attention to women in labour. There are no other duties to be performed. She is not responsible for a hospital ward nor for an operating theatre in the event of caesarean section. She wears a distinctive uniform so that she can be instantly recognized. Without doubt her greatest reward is the tremendous sense of job satisfaction that she derives from the ability to make such a worthwhile contribution to the resolution of the age-old problem of stress in labour on what truly could be described as a grand scale. Among the many benefits that have come from the practice of Active Management of Labour, none is more gratifying to observe than the boost given to the professional status of nurses.

Staff Nurse-Midwife

A staff nurse acts as an assistant to the sister-in-charge of the delivery unit and is responsible directly to her. Two staff nurses are present at all times and their hours of duty correspond to those of the sister-in-charge. A staff nurse, like a sister-in-charge, acts in a supervisory capacity and in normal circumstances is not identified with an individual patient. At least one trained midwife is present at every delivery, and she conducts most deliveries herself.

Pupil Nurse-Midwife

Five pupils complete the team. A pupil plays a different role. She provides continuous support for one woman throughout labour. This role ensures that she comes to appreciate that a nurse's unique contribution to the management of labour is made at personal level. This requires that far more attention be paid to a woman's face than to her uterus or to vital signs. As this is a teaching hospital, pupils perform these duties, which would be suitable for trained midwives elsewhere.

The actual procedure is as follows: a woman is admitted to the delivery unit by a pupil, who remains with her throughout labour, conducts her delivery, presents her newborn infant and eventually accompanies her to a postnatal ward. This ideal is not always realized in full because it is affected by hours of duty, but as labour rarely lasts longer than eight hours it applies in most cases. It is very seldom indeed that more than two nurses are involved consecutively with the same patient. Each nurse appreciates that it is her primary duty to sustain her patient's flagging spirits during the tedious hours of the first stage of labour and then encourage her to achieve spontaneous delivery through her own efforts in the second stage.

Each pupil spends almost six months in the delivery unit during the total period of two years required for midwifery training.

General Principles

The personal nurse is advised to sit always in front of and in direct eye contact with a recumbent patient, not to stand over her in a dominant position, and never behind her out of her line of vision. A comfortable seat is provided for this purpose. Should a woman prefer to walk, her nurse walks too.

Nurses are encouraged to develop close personal relationships with mothers and to converse with them on any subject that holds their interest, thus distracting attention from the labour predicament. In our experience young properly motivated girls perform this task with remarkable success when they are made sufficiently conscious of the need and given the right example by their superiors. Nurses are taught that women in labour have a natural tendency to withdraw from contact with their surroundings and turn inwards on themselves, and that this inclination to introspection is greatly exaggerated by analgesic drugs. They are forewarned about the woman who closes her eyes, buries her face in the pillow and continues to complain even between contractions. They know these are signs that indicate that the thread of personal contact is being broken and that once broken it will be very difficult to mend. They are acutely sensitive to the fact that a woman who turns her back passes a devastating judgement on the quality of the nursing care.

Two subjects of conversation that are of abiding interest to every woman in labour are the expected time of delivery and the welfare of her unborn child. A good nurse appreciates that her patient needs constant reassurance that she is making steady progress and that her baby is likely to be born soon. This information should be instantly available on every worthwhile partograph. Hopefully the graph will have been explained beforehand, at antenatal classes, with this important sequel in mind. In this case mothers can be expected to take a keen interest in the medical proceedings. A partograph that does not fulfil a predictive function loses much of its value.

Specific Duties

The personal nurse has specific clinical duties to perform at regular intervals during labour. She must record the mother's pulse, temperature, respirations, blood pressure and urine, together with the fetal heart and liquor. In the event of oxytocin being used, she must regulate the rate of infusion and record each contraction. She works under close supervision and must report any untoward event to her superiors.

Summary

No form of management in labour can be really effective unless it can be practised by nurses almost independently of doctors. This requires a level of confidence, between nurses and doctors, which is not too often found. A clear chain of command that can be seen to function with near military efficiency but always with a human face is an essential requirement. Nurses and doctors must become accustomed to the viewpoint that much more can be contributed to the emotional stability of mothers than to their physical welfare in circumstances where some 95% are normal at the point of admission.

One of the most impressive features of Active Management of Labour is the sense of genuine purpose that it gives to all members of the nursing profession who work in a busy delivery unit.

22

Role of the Mother

It could all too easily be overlooked that mothers themselves have the most important contribution to make to labour. No matter how high the quality of care on offer from nurses and doctors, the entire experience can well prove disastrous when the mother is not properly prepared. Therefore a serious obligation rests on expectant mothers to take full advantage of the educational facilities available so as to learn the nature of their role and how best this may be fulfilled. Mothers should not be allowed—any more than nurses or doctors are allowed—to evade their responsibilities in this matter. They should be disabused of the notion that nurses and doctors can be expected to cope with the situation as part of their normal duties. Paternalism is not to be considered a virtue here and an expectant mother should be made to face the fact that the birth of her child is primarily her responsibility.

All this, of course, is to suppose that adequate educational facilities are readily available and relevant in content. Above all, what is taught must be seen to correspond with events that take place in that institution. Not only must teachers be credible, but nurses and doctors who care for women in labour must know exactly what they have been taught. If more than lip service is to be paid to the proposition that education is a necessary component of an obstetric service with pretensions to acceptable standards of care in labour, then classes must cease to be regarded as optional extras conducted by teachers who are far removed from clinical practice and virtually ignored by those in positions of greatest influence. The most important element in the whole educational process is education to the need for education, and only clinicians are in a position to impress this on their patients. It is much too late to begin education in labour.

Every adult woman must, in the final analysis, be made to feel the proper custodian of her own well-being, not to mention that of her child. Labour is no exception to this general rule. An expectant mother owes it to herself, her husband and her child, and to every other woman who shares the facilities of the delivery unit, to be well briefed on the subject of a mothers contribution to labour. This disruptive effect of one disorganized and frightened woman in a delivery unit extends far beyond her own comfort and safety, and there should be no hesitation in telling her so.

Mothers also have a duty to those who care for them in labour. The reciprocal nature of this contract deserves much more emphasis than it has been given. Where necessary it should be clearly stated that nurses are not expected to submit themselves to the sometimes outrageous conduct of perfectly healthy women who could not be persuaded to cross a corridor from an antenatal clinic to learn how to behave with dignity and purpose during the most important event of their lives. Nor should nurses be held responsible for the degrading scenes that occasionally result from the failure of a woman to fulfil her part of the contract.

Women who have participated in the educational programme of this hospital generally portray a high level of insight into the essential features of the birth process. They understand the need for professional confirmation of their provisional diagnosis of labour, they know that progress is measured in terms of the opening of the neck of the womb, and when progress is slow they appreciate that it makes good sense to take corrective action on time. All this is evident from the partograph, with which they are already familiar. Not surprisingly, therefore, women in labour often request acceleration with oxytocin when it becomes clear that progress is not being made. By way of contrast, they require to be convinced whenever the question of induction is mooted.

Suggestions that women in some other centres regard oxytocin with suspicion and in the event of slow progress not infrequently decline acceleration can only be the result of misunderstandings, which reflect poorly on the quality of the educational service. Paradoxically, induction rates that involve identical procedures may be close to 50% in these same centres. Time and again the authors are impressed by the ability of the average woman to assimilate the essential facts about labour when these are properly presented.

Summary

Expectant mothers deserve to be treated as adults and made fully aware that childbirth is primarily their responsibility. But they must be provided with adequate educational services so that they can learn to deliver their own infants. Obstetricians must realize that few adult women really wish to be treated as irresponsible children.

23

Care of the Fetus

Overall care of the fetus during labour is based on the simple premise that the fetus who presents as a case of hypoxia during the course of normal labour is almost sure to have been embarrassed before labour began. The occasional exception is likely to be the result of an accident of labour, which causes acute hypoxia in a hitherto normal fetus: prolapse of cord is the classical example. The aims of care of the fetus, therefore, are twofold: first, to identify the fetus who is already embarrassed; and second, to ensure that labour remains normal.[11]

Artificial Rupture of Membranes

To identify the fetus who is already embarrassed, artificial rupture of membranes is performed as soon as a formal diagnosis of labour has been made and the woman is therefore committed to delivery. A free flow of clear liquor is regarded as a virtual guarantee that the function of the placenta is sufficient to withstand the pressures of normal labour. The opportunity is taken to exclude prolapse of cord. A sample of liquor is retained for subsequent inspection in every case.

This procedure is intended to identify the cases that have escaped detection in late pregnancy before the additional stress of labour can cause an already precarious balance to deteriorate rapidly.

Meconium

Meconium is regarded as a clinical sign of great potential significance. At the outset women in labour are divided into two groups: some 90% with clear liquor and 10% with meconium. The division into low-risk and high-risk cases is made on this evidence, which is of fetal origin, and not on whether, for example, the mother suffers from pre-eclampsia or had her last menstruation 42 weeks previously.

Not all meconium, however, is accorded the same significance. There is a world of difference between light meconium staining of a large volume of liquor and meconium that is virtually undiluted, with umbilical cord, membranes and even endometrium coloured green through its entire depth when subsequently exposed at caesarean section.

Meconium is regarded as evidence of placental insufficiency of some considerable duration and not as evidence of short-term fetal distress. Moreover, meconium seldom appears for the first time during the course of normal labour.

Three grades of meconium are recognized, as follows:

Grade I   —A good volume of liquor, lightly stained with meconium.
Grade II —A reasonable volume of liquor, with a heavy suspension of meconium.
Grade III—Thick meconium, which is undiluted and resembles sieved spinach.

All grades of meconium must be reported to the senior resident on duty. A wide margin of discretion is permitted in Grade I, and after careful review of the clinical circumstances, no further action is taken in most cases. A fetal blood sample is mandatory in Grade II, and treatment is determined largely by the result. Caesarean section is performed in Grade III unless an easy vaginal delivery is imminent; as not only hypoxia but also meconium inhalation is a real possibility here.

No Liquor

Failure to recover any liquor whatsoever at artificial rupture of membrane is, for reasons of safety, treated as meconium Grade II, although clear liquor frequently appears at a later stage.

Fetal Heart

Direct auscultation of the fetal heart is a duty performed by the personal nurse, who supervises each individual in labour. This is for one full minute, at intervals of 15 minutes during the first stage and after each contraction during the second stage.

Blood Sample

Fetal acidosis is accepted as the definitive test for hypoxia. Only in exceptional circumstances is a woman subjected to caesarean section for the indication fetal distress without this confirmation. In practice, this situation is likely to arise mainly in the case of Grade II meconium, where caesarean section would have to be performed—sometimes unnecessarily—were the test not available.

Electronic Monitors

Electronic monitors do not play a part in the routine care of the fetus in this hospital. But in the event of a blood sample being taken because of clinical evidence of distress—most likely in the form of meconium at rupture of membranes—a scalp electrode is applied before the result is known. This ensures a continuous record between definitive blood tests in suspect cases, but it would be highly improbable that the tracing would, of itself, determine treatment.

Because of the still unsettled controversy concerning the respective values of continuous electronic monitoring and intermittent auscultation, a decision was made to compare the two methods in the context of the practice of this hospital. Arising from this, a randomized trial of unprecedented scope was undertaken by our colleague Dr Dermot MacDonald and members of staff, in conjunction with the National Perinatal Epidemiology Unit in the United Kingdom, between March 1981 and April 1983. Specifically excluded from the trial beforehand were cases with meconium or no liquor at rupture of membranes; these represented 6% of the total. All other cases, without regard to risk status by conventional standards like pre-eclampsia, antepartum haemorrhage, diabetes, etc., were included. The number of eligible cases was 13 025, of which 6474 were allocated on a random basis to the electronically monitored group and 6490 to the intermittently auscultated group. Both methods were supported by fetal blood samples as the need arose. The results showed no difference in perinatal mortality rate: there were 14 deaths in each group. Neither was there a significant difference in Apgar scores, need for intubation or admission to the Special Care Baby Unit. There was, however, one significant difference: the incidence of neonatal convulsions in those who survived. There were nine cases of neonatal convulsions in the electronically monitored group, compared with 21 in the intermittently auscultated group. When these 30 infants were examined after 12 months, six showed evidence of permanent damage, all of the cerebral palsy type: three were from the electronically monitored group and three from the intermittently auscultated group. The balance, in other words, had been restored. These children will be reviewed at regular intervals over an indefinite period of time.[16,17]

Incidentally, the perinatal mortality rate in the cases excluded from the trial on the basis of meconium or no liquor was five times greater than the overall figure for the cases included. The caesarean section rate was low and not significantly different in either group, at 2.4 and 2.2%, respectively. Elective caesarean sections are, of course, not represented. The close similarity between the groups is almost certainly the result of retaining the blood sample as the final arbiter of distress in both instances, as there can be little doubt that electronic monitors without the benefit of blood tests as control lead to a sharp increase in the caesarean section rate for the indication of fetal distress.

Normal Labour

Since the contention is that normal placental function is sufficient to sustain the fetus through the exigencies of normal labour, it is necessary to have a clear understanding of what is meant by this term. Labour is defined as normal when delivery is effected within 12 hours mainly through the efforts of the mother, although this need not exclude the use of low forceps. Steps taken to ensure that labour conforms to this definition of normality would appear to be a valuable contribution to the welfare of the fetus also. Of course, trauma must be avoided at all costs and is much less likely to occur when mothers deliver themselves.

Summary

A fetus who enters labour in good condition is by nature well equipped to withstand the challenge of normal birth. Routine supervision in this hospital is based on simple clinical evidence, meticulously observed. Particular attention is paid to meconium present at the outset. This evidence is universally available and needs no specialized techniques. Electronic monitors represent an alternative method of routine supervision. In either event a fetal blood sample serves to reduce the caesarean section rate for the indication fetal distress.

24

Induction

This manual is not concerned with induction as a separate issue, but only indirectly in so far as induction may impinge on management of labour. The subject was discussed briefly in Chapter 2, in which two points were emphatically made: first, that there must be no confusion between induction and acceleration of labour; and second, that induction has a profoundly adverse effect on management of labour in general. The adverse effects of induction are by no means confined to the individuals directly involved but extend to everyone delivered in a hospital in which induction is freely practised. Against this background there are three different aspects of the subject that merit close attention: (i) indications for induction; (ii) suitability for induction; and (iii) method of induction.[9]

Indications

The looseness or otherwise of the indications for induction determines the size of the iatrogenic problem created by this form of medical intervention in each institution. One of the many adverse effects of an uncritical application of statistics to obstetric practice in recent years has been to extend the indications for induction to include almost everyone. Pre-eclampsia and prolonged pregnancy are the two outstanding examples, because these are the indications for induction recorded in the great majority of cases, whether the incidence be high or low. While it is true that pre-eclampsia and prolonged pregnancy are both associated with a significant increase in perinatal mortality, this applies only when the diastolic pressure exceeds 100 mm or the duration of pregnancy exceeds 42 weeks. The statistics have been widely misinterpreted, with the result that a high proportion of all patients on whom induction is performed for pre-eclampsia or prolonged pregnancy—or some equally vague reason—do not conform to critical standards. Furthermore, even in the minority who do conform to critical standards, the likelihood of an unfavourable outcome is so small that it does not justify a routine approach, where many are subjected to a potentially dangerous form of treatment in the hope that a few may benefit. Induction of labour, so called, is undertaken much too often on a rule of thumb basis, with little attempt to select the individuals who are genuinely in need of deliverance.

In this hospital indications for induction are becoming increasingly selective, as for example in pre-eclampsia and post-maturity, which together account for the bulk of reported cases everywhere. Induction is now rarely performed for pre-eclampsia unless in addition to hypertension there is proteinuria, or for post-maturity unless there is objective evidence of impaired placental function, as shown by reduced liquor volume at ultrasound examination at 42 weeks. The general conclusion is that the rate of induction overall should not exceed 10%, which represents about 800 women per annum in this hospital.

Suitability

The standard of suitability adopted largely determines the number of failures. As the indication for delivery is seldom absolute, the decision to proceed with induction should be subject to the likelihood of success in each individual case. Induction is not attempted in this hospital unless the baby's head is engaged and the cervix at least reasonably favourable. Whenever the need to terminate pregnancy arises before these basic conditions are fulfilled caesarean section is usually performed, on the grounds that induction is not the correct method of treatment. Prostaglandin to ripen the cervix is seldom considered appropriate in these circumstances. Attention is drawn to the fact that the overall incidence of caesarean section is less than 5% in spite of this apparently radical approach.

The suggestion, which is not infrequently made (at least by implication) that the end justifies the means in this context, and that whatever happens later can be blamed on the condition for which the induction was nominally performed, is simply not tenable. In all walks of life prudence requires that no action be taken without due consideration of the possible consequences and this is certainly true of obstetrics also. The decision to interrupt the course of pregnancy is a classic example of a balance of risks. A decision to embark on induction as the method of achieving this end may be quite correct in one instance, because the conditions are favourable, but incorrect in another, because the conditions are unfavourable. Far too many inductions are undertaken for questionable reasons, in unfavourable circumstances, with the result that the treatment is more dangerous than the often nebulous disease. An uncritical approach to this potentially serious matter is the cause of considerable disquiet, which is not confined to obstetricians.

Method

The method of induction determines the time spent in a delivery unit by women who are not yet in labour. This consideration has very important implications, both for the individuals directly involved and for all other women passing through the delivery unit, especially where there is a large number of inductions. To reduce the time spent in the delivery unit by women not yet in labour—primarily in their own interest, but also in the interest of others—the method of induction used in this hospital consists of simple amniotomy. The final decision to proceed with amniotomy is taken at pelvic examination by a doctor with the status of senior resident. The forewaters are ruptured in a different location and at a fixed time of day. The woman returns to the antenatal ward to await the onset of labour. Meanwhile, no restrictions are placed on her movements. The result is that 90% of women subjected to amniotomy for the purpose of induction are already in labour when they enter the delivery unit. Subsequent progress is the same in all respects as in women admitted from their homes, whether expressed in terms of hours spent in the delivery unit, drugs administered for the relief of pain, or the number of operative procedures performed.

Labour does not begin within 24 hours of amniotomy in 10% of cases. These are recorded as failed inductions. They are transferred to the delivery unit next morning and oxytocin is given as a back-up procedure. The solution used, which is the same as for acceleration of labour, is 10 units in one litre of 5% dextrose. The maximum rate of infusion is 60 drops per minute and only one litre is allowed. The result is that 90% of these cases, already classified as failed induction because they did not respond to simple amniotomy, deliver vaginally within 12 hours. Caesarean section is performed when labour is not well advanced after one litre, which takes about six hours, or when a woman has been 12 hours in the delivery unit.

This method of procedure ensures that only one woman in every 100 admitted to the delivery unit of this hospital receives oxytocin for the purpose of induction; in numerical terms this means 80 women out of a total of some 8000 on an annual basis. The contribution made by this simple arrangement to the overall quality of care afforded to the 8000 women in labour is enormous. The facilities, especially in terms of human resources, are not dissipated in the care of women not in labour and who a priori should therefore not be in a delivery unit. There are many delivery units in which, at any one time, half of all the women are not in labour. Yet these are the very women who attract most attention and for a much longer time. This level of attention can only be made available at the expense of the women who are in labour.

The main argument advanced in support of the immediate use of oxytocin to induce labour after amniotomy is based on the fact that the likelihood of infection increases with the time that elapses between amniotomy and delivery: the induction–delivery interval. In practice, however, the risk is small when cases are carefully selected and delivery is almost sure to take place within 24 hours. Under these circumstances the risk of infection is certainly not sufficient to justify serious disruption of an entire delivery unit by the admission of a large number of women who are not in labour. This is an example of the balance of risks applied to a wider issue.

Summary

The impact of a hospital policy that involves a high rate of induction cannot be evaluated in isolation. It is not sufficient to examine the immediate results of induction itself, the indirect effects on all other aspects of practice must also be taken into account. The adverse effects of a high rate of induction on the overall management of labour are so great that it might reasonably be argued that the greatest single contribution to improved standards of care in labour would be a virtual embargo on this procedure. As a complete embargo is not a practical proposition, induction should be regarded as a necessary evil, to be restricted to a small number of cases in which the indication is genuine and the conditions are favourable. The method should be chosen to cause the least disturbance to the individual and the least disruption to the delivery unit. Unquestionably, simple amniotomy is the method: only one woman in every 100 receives oxytocin to induce labour in this hospital, yet the caesarean section rate is less than 5%.

25

Organization

Although, no doubt, there are many other fields of medical practice of which it could be said with equal truth that there is more to be gained from sound organizational methods than from sophisticated techniques, there can be few more obvious examples than a modern delivery unit. No matter how sophisticated the equipment may become a delivery unit cannot begin to function properly unless the basic organization is sound.[4]

Delivery units generally suffer from poor organizational standards mainly because they lack central direction, and, in management terms often border on the chaotic because they are unable to cope with occasional pressures, although overstaffed for most of the time. Corporate spirit is often poorly developed, with nurses, doctors and even administrators failing to co-operate with one another when not actually in open conflict, sometimes within the same group. Inevitably this is to the detriment of the entire service.

Better organization can literally transform the quality of care provided for all women in labour; it can enhance the level of job satisfaction of nurses and provide an objective basis for the economics involved in a very expensive service. As is so often the case in medicine, good practice corresponds with good economics in this instance. Both make sense.

Nursing Services

In terms of organization, the key to the solution of the problems of a modern delivery unit lies in nursing services. Nursing staff must be deployed for the declared purpose of providing professional attention at a personal level for every woman in labour. The same number of nurses of equal status must operate day and night as clear testimony to the fact that the welfare of mothers and infants is not to be adversely affected by the time at which a birth happens to occur. This cannot be achieved through a haphazard approach: careful planning is needed.

Scale

A large-scale operation is an obvious advantage because it helps to eliminate peaks and troughs in terms of babies born at different hours of the day, or days of the week or seasons of the year. In this hospital, with some 8000 deliveries per annum, the percentage of total births that occurs in each of the

8-hour periods corresponding with official working shifts falls between 30 and 35, and in each month of the year between 7.5 and 9.5. This provides a reasonably even distribution. Furthermore, scale permits a nucleus of highly-skilled nurses to be employed on a whole-time basis in the delivery unit so that they are not required to divide their attention between antenatal and postnatal wards, nor leave women in labour to assist at caesarean sections.

Intensive Care

Nowadays delivery units are frequently spoken of in the context of intensive care units, in spite of the fact that services, especially nursing services, continue to function on an ad hoc basis, devoid of any rational explanation and heavily concentrated in daylight hours, to suit staff rather than patients, it would appear. There is a yawning credibility gap here that needs to be closed.

Bottleneck

The delivery unit represents a bottleneck in every maternity hospital, through which all mothers must pass, and it is here that the number of confinements that it is possible to cater for in the system is determined. Accommodation elsewhere, especially in postnatal wards, which comprise the bulk of obstetrical beds, is extremely flexible. The immediate effect of a general reduction of stay in a postnatal ward by one day would be to increase the functional capacity of a maternity hospital by at least 20%. These are considerations of great practical importance in terms of public expenditure at current levels. Only a special care baby unit can compare with a delivery unit in terms of concentration of skill and corresponding costs. Both should be efficiently used. Antenatal and postnatal wards are areas of comparatively low level care, where most mothers can and indeed should fend for themselves.

Duration of Stay

The newfound ability to limit the duration of stay and therefore to quantify the number of patient-hours to be serviced has transformed the previously haphazard approach to planning for labour. To take a simple example: one nurse in the course of a working day can supervise one woman during a labour that lasts eight hours, whereas three nurses are required to supervise the same woman during a labour lasting 24 hours. Of course, the problem is greatly compounded by the extensive use of induction, where nurses are engaged in looking after patients who for much of the time are not in labour. A liberal policy towards induction constitutes an almost insurmountable barrier to the application of sound organizational methods in a delivery unit, especially where the all-important matter of nursing services is concerned.

The Practice

There were 7853 babies born in the National Maternity Hospital during 1984. The total nursing complement employed in the delivery unit was 40, of whom 19 were trained and 21 were pupil midwives. This number includes provision for holiday relief and other off-duty situations, such as study leave and occasional illness. There was no other category of nursing attendant involved. Hence the number of babies born for every nurse employed was 196. This compares with 207 in 1970, when 6225 babies were born. The latter was the subject of a report in the *Proceedings of the Royal Society of Medicine*.[4] At that time comparison was made with the average figure of 84 births per nurse employed in the delivery unit in a sample of five similar hospitals around the British Isles. The unit cost of production, relating salaries paid to nurses to the number of babies born, was three times as high in the other hospitals, although remuneration was at the same level. Paradoxically, this was the only hospital of the six surveyed where a personal nurse was provided for everyone in labour.

Nurses work eight-hour shifts. The number of nurses on duty in the delivery unit at all times is eight: one sister-in-charge, two staff nurses and five student nurses. There are five delivery rooms. To ensure that everyone in labour has continuous personal attention, one student nurse is allotted to each room. Staff nurses act in a supervisory capacity, with the sister in complete charge. A sister-in-charge or staff nurse employed in the delivery unit works 33 hours and 36 minutes, and a student nurse 40 hours each week. Hence the unit cost of production, in which nurses' salaries are by far the largest item, can be readily estimated. This provides a basis of comparison from year to year and between one institution and another. Owing to a steady decline in total births from a peak of 8964 in 1981, the number of deliveries per nurse employed fell below the critical figure of 200 in 1984 for the first time. Steps have since been taken to restore the balance.

Although none is as important as the nursing element, there are several other aspects of the total organizational requirement of an efficient delivery service, which hopefully may have been discerned as a continuous thread running through the pages of this book. Most important of all is the need for central direction which will draw the diverse elements together, creating a team out of a number of individuals of various disciplines and different levels of seniority, a result that is reflected in an efficient, happy and economical unit, which can be seen to make sense to all who work there.

Summary

The ideal combination of a nucleus of highly skilled nurses with continuous personal attention for every woman in labour is feasible in a busy unit only where a limit is set to the duration of labour and everyone receives individual attention simply because it is needed for a shorter time. But it would be naive in the extreme to assume that this situation could be achieved overnight or that it is simply a matter of opting for the correct technical procedures. In the final analysis, good organization is more important to labour management than any number of sophisticated techniques.

26

The Cervix in Labour

Obstetrics suffers grievously from lack of definition not only the common clinical conditions of which labour is itself a prime example but also of the terms currently used to describe various aspects of these conditions. One suspects that were several individuals working in the same delivery unit and accustomed to exchanging these familiar terms every day asked what precisely they understood the words 'effacement' and 'dilatation' to mean, or, better still, were they presented with a pencil and paper and asked to reproduce them in a visual way, the results would be very different. Yet hardly anyone would dispute that it is a matter of considerable practical consequence that there should be at least a common language amongst co-workers in the field.

Parity Factor

Time and again in the preceding chapters attention has been drawn to the need to consider primigravidae and multigravidae as if they belonged to different biological species, particularly in all matters relating to labour. The cervix is one more example. To the examining finger, the primigravid cervix and the multigravid cervix are so dissimilar that they could well be different organs. The greatest divergence concerns the external os, which remains permanently open after the birth of a first child. This is a source of endless confusion. The parity factor must be taken into account whenever the terms 'effacement' and 'dilatation' are under consideration. The best way to illustrate this is by diagrammatic representation:

The nulliparous cervix is tubular in shape and although constricted somewhat at either end, both internal os and external os usually allow a fingertip to pass.

The parous cervix is tent-like in shape with an internal os of comparable size but an external os that hangs loose to the extent that it may allow two fingers or more to pass.

Effacement

Effacement refers to the process of inclusion of the length of the cervical canal into the lower segment or body of the uterus. This begins at the internal os and proceeds downwards to the external os, at which level effacement is complete. The process of effacement is not tied to a particular time schedule: it may occur late in pregnancy or be delayed in its entirety until labour begins. An important corollary to this is that effacement of the cervix is not an essential requirement for a diagnosis of labour: a woman may well be in labour without her cervix being effaced, much less dilated. Hence the practical importance of a 'show' or spontaneous rupture of membranes, as discussed in Chapter 5. But in the event of effacement not having taken place at least to some extent beforehand, the duration of labour is likely to be prolonged. These are usually the troublesome cases.

Dilatation

Dilatation refers to the external os only. The external os cannot begin to open until the process of effacement is complete. Effacement and dilatation are consecutive not simultaneous events. This sequential relationship is of paramount importance: a cervix that is not effaced cannot be dilated, even though, as is often the case in a parous woman, the external os freely admits two fingers at pelvic examination. The patulous state of the external os in a parous woman is a consequence of a previous birth; passive in nature, it must not be confused with the active process of dilatation, which denotes labour here and now. Naturally, by the time a parous cervix achieves full effacement it is already the equivalent of 2 cm on the dilatation scale.

Transition

The point of transition at which effacement ends and dilatation begins requires special attention. At this point, presence or absence of painful uterine contractions is decisive. Because without painful uterine contractions there is no possibility of a woman being in labour, a fully-effaced cervix in these circumstances should be said to admit one or more fingers, as the case may be, whereas with painful uterine contractions the same cervix should be said to be dilated to the extent of one or more centimetres. The former expression is intended to convey an inert or static situation, while the latter is intended to convey an evolving or dynamic situation. At a practical level the issue is simple: should an individual who believes herself to be in labour be retained in the delivery unit, with the almost inevitable consequence that she is committed to delivery, perhaps ultimately by caesarean section? As one caesarean section may well lead to another, the woman's lifestyle may be significantly altered as a result of this decision. Hence the need for close attention to detail in this pivotal area. (See Figure 2.)

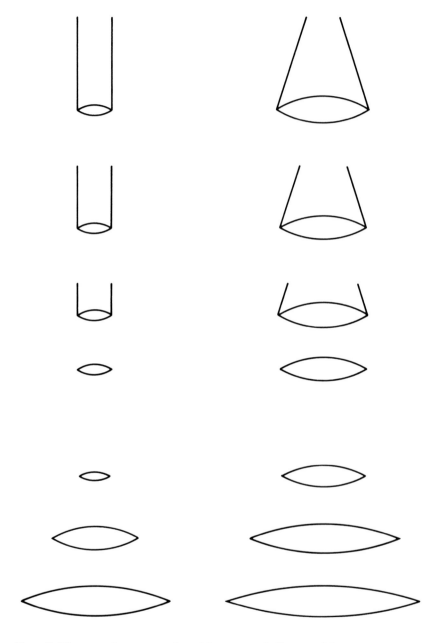

Figure 2. Diagrammatic representation of the process of effacement followed by dilatation of the primigravid and of the multigravid cervix.

Summary

There is nowhere sufficient appreciation of the fact that very many of the problems encountered in a delivery unit have their origin in wrong diagnosis. Unwittingly, these are classified under the heading dystocia or one of its three subsidiaries: inefficient uterine action, posterior position or cephalopelvic disproportion. Given the fundamental importance of diagnosis and of the central role of the cervix in the decision-making process, surprisingly little attention is directed to the perceived meaning of the terms used to describe the sequence of events that occur at this critical juncture. Instead, the terms 'effacement' and 'dilatation' tend to be taken for granted and quickly glossed over, as if everybody understood clearly what they meant. As always, the need for verbal precision is greatest in the doubtful cases where diagnosis presents a genuine problem; no such problem arises when the cervix is well dilatated, and these cases give rise to few difficulties during the course of labour in any case.

27

Caesarean Section Rates

There can be very little doubt that from the maternal aspect of childbirth, at least, the most striking change in the practice of obstetrics over the past 20 years is the explosive growth in caesarean section almost everywhere. The caesarean birth-rate across the USA increased fourfold—from 5 to 20%— between 1965 and 1980, representing a numerical increase from 150 000 to 600 000 annually. Similar trends have been reported from Canada, South America, Australia, Western Europe and Scandinavia, and increasingly from less developed countries open to Western influence. Whether calculated in terms of human anxiety and discomfort, of surgical and anaesthetic complications, which, although usually minor, are sometimes major and occasionally fatal, or in purely monetary terms, the cost is truly enormous[13].

Sense of Proportion

In the light of the extraordinary increase in the number of women subjected to abdominal operations that are of no direct benefit to themselves, the detached observer might reasonably assume that the benefits conferred on their offspring could be shown to be overwhelming. But that is far from being the case. Indeed, Pearson, writing in the *American Journal of Obstetrics and Gynecology* in January 1984, described the phenomenon as the greatest uncontrolled medical experiment of our time. As justification for the increase in the caesarean section rate must be sought in improved perinatal results, the tables presented in Section III of this manual are of particular interest; similar information is not readily available from other sources. Briefly, the tables show that at 4.2%, the caesarean section rate has not changed over 20 years, while the perinatal mortality rate has declined from 36 to 12 per thousand over the same period of time. These figures provide a basis for comparison with other centres.

An increase of just 1% in the caesarean section rate at this hospital would entail 80 additional operations, 5% would entail 400 additional operations, and 10% would entail 800 additional operations, on an annual basis. At a practical level this would mean that at least two additional caesarean sections would be performed on each day of the year. As most would be at irregular hours, this would create a logistical problem of major proportions, which could be resolved only to the detriment of other services. And still the caesarean section rate would not exceed 15%, a figure that seems perfectly

108

acceptable in many comparable establishments. So much for the mother, what of the child?

In 1984 there were 91 perinatal deaths in this hospital (12 per 1000), of which 40 (5 per 1000) were the result of lethal congenital malformation. Among 51 (7 per 1000) normal infants, 13 (1.7 per 1000) were alive when labour began, and of these, eight (1 per 1000) died during labour and five (0.7 per 1000) during the seven days after birth. The last figure is a fine tribute to our colleagues in neonatology, but it hardiy supports a case for the extended use of caesarean section. There is no acceptable standard for comparison in the 7762 (988 per 1000) infants who survived, but Paneth and Stark, in an epidemiological overview of cerebral palsy and mental deficiency in relation to indicators of perinatal asphyxia in New York City, in the *American Journal of Obstetrics and Gynecology*, December 1983, concluded that 'obstetric intervention based solely on concern for later neurological development cannot be justified'.

Impact of Neonatology

The general reduction in perinatal mortality in recent years coincided with the emergence of neonatology as a major speciality, thus leading to the present position, where given a normal infant born alive without hypoxia or trauma after 28 weeks, or even less in a tertiary care centre, it is almost sure to survive and, hopefully, to develop satisfactorily. The very success of neonatologists has resulted in subtle pressure being brought to bear on obstetricians to dispense with the whole wearisome process of labour altogether. This would seem a perfectly reasonable proposition were there only one patient to be considered. But unfortunately in obstetrics there are two, and while no one would dispute the contention that babies have a right to be wellborn, experience compiled in this hospital over an extended period shows that similar results can be achieved by far less intrusive means. Whenever the occasion arises, therefore, it is a matter of the utmost importance that facile conclusions in respect of cause and effect between caesarean section rates and perinatal mortality rates, much less morbidity rates, should be challenged; otherwise, it is not inconceivable that eventually all babies will be born by caesarean section, if only because obstetricians are forced into a position of having to protect themselves from charges of malpractice. Mothers will be the losers if obstetricians renege on the dual responsibility that is the distinctive feature of their speciality. (See Figure 3.)

Indications

The National Institutes of Health Consensus Development Report on Cesarean Childbirth* clearly identifies dystocia (abnormal labour) as the

---

*US Department of Health and Human Services, Public Health Service, National Institutes of Health Publication No. 82–2067, October 1981.

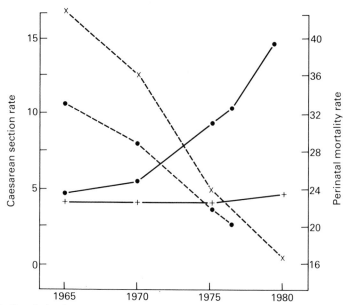

Figure 3. Correlation between caesarean and perinatal mortality rates. Caesarean section rates per 100 deliveries are represented by solid lines and perinatal mortality rates per 1000 deliveries by broken lines: in the National Maternity Hospital, Dublin (crosses)[13] and in the United States according to Bottoms, S. F., Rosen, M. G. & Dokol, R. J. (1980) The increase in the caesarean birth rate. *New England Journal of Medicine* 302: 559–563.

main reason for the expansion of caesarean section in the USA. Dystocia accounts for one in two of all primary operations and, by inference, for at least the same proportion of repeat procedures. The low caesarean section rate in this hospital can be explained almost entirely by the figure for dystocia. The caesarean section rate for dystocia alone in the USA exceeds

Indications for Caesarean Section
(expressed as a percentage of all births)

	USA* (1978)	Dublin† (1984)
Abnormal labour	4.7	0.5
Repeat	4.7	1.1
Breech	1.8	0.5
Fetal distress	0.8	0.4
Others	3.2	1.7
	15.2	4.2

*NIH Consensus Report.
†National Maternity Hospital.

the caesarean section rate for all indications in Dublin. There are differences under other headings, such as fetal distress and breech presentation, but these are small by comparison. Ultimately, the caesarean section rate anywhere is determined by the management of labour in first-time mothers with a vertex presentation and single fetus, which is what this book is about. Parous women do not suffer from dystocia to any significant extent.

Caesarean section rates were not a factor taken into account when the original decision was taken to improve the quality of care extended to all women in labour in this hospital. They were not an issue 20 years ago, being much the same everywhere. The low caesarean section rates that have continued in this hospital through the intervening years must be seen as testimony to the fundamental truth that efficient uterine action is the key to normal labour. Meanwhile, and for the same reason, the duration of labour has been restricted and traumatic vaginal delivery in the form of rotational forceps has been eliminated[15].

Counting the Cost

Given the lack of evidence that the massive increase in caesarean section rates throughout much of the Western world has resulted in any tangible benefits for infants, there are several pertinent questions to be asked. Does it really matter what the caesarean section rate is in a particular hospital or community? At an individual level, is it a matter of any great consequence that a woman's first baby is delivered by caesarean section, possibly under epidural anaesthesia, with her husband present and given that she is not likely to have more than two children in any event? For the obstetrician who carries a dual responsibility, are there considerations of professional ethics in so far as the mother's welfare is concerned? Who created the medicolegal climate that is said to be a factor in many countries and dominant in some? What are the repercussions of this change in practice on the Third World, from where so many graduates are trained in Western methods? Sooner or later these questions will have to be answered; they cannot be avoided as caesarean section rates continue to rise.

Summary

There has been an unwarranted increase in the caesarean birth-rate in many countries in recent years. Most of the additional operations are performed on normal women—primigravidae with a vertex presentation and single fetus—for the indication dystocia. Inevitably, the more primary sections performed today, the more secondary sections will be necessary tomorrow. As effective uterine action is the key to normal labour, the central problem of dystocia can be solved by much simpler means. A caesarean section rate of 4.2% in this hospital in 1984 is a direct result.

SECTION II
Visual Records of Labour

Primigravid Labour

PRIMIGRAVID LABOUR

A sharp distinction is drawn between first and subsequent labour because the causes of delay and the risks of treatment are very different.

Slow progress is common in primigravidae and is almost always an expression of inefficient uterine action, whereas slow progress is uncommon in multigravidae and when it occurs is frequently an expression of obstruction. Obstruction is caused by a fetal complication such as malpresentation or malformation, that is hydrocephalus. Similarly, oxytocin does not cause rupture of the primigravid uterus even in the presence of cephalopelvic disproportion, whereas oxytocin may cause rupture of the multigravid uterus even in normal circumstances. This is one of the fundamental truths of clinical obstetrics, on which Active Management of Labour is based.

To ensure that this distinction is maintained at all times, the Primigravid Labour Record is printed on a yellow background and the Multigravid Labour Record is printed on a blue background. This simple innovation has proved to be of enormous value in the everyday practice of this hospital and it is strongly recommended to others, because failure to make the distinction between primigravidae and multigravidae is the main cause of misunderstanding in the management of labour.

All of the charts that follow are yellow save one and therefore refer to primigravidae; this is a measure of the importance attached to first labour.

GRAPH 1

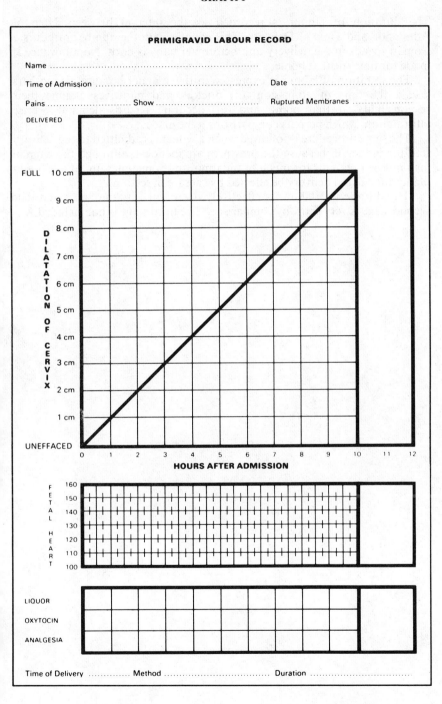

PRIMIGRAVID LABOUR RECORD

Name ....

Time of Admission .... Date ....

Pains .... Show .... Ruptured Membranes ....

DELIVERED

FULL   10 cm

9 cm

8 cm

D
I
L   7 cm
A
T   6 cm
A
T
I   5 cm
O
N   4 cm
O
F   3 cm
C
E   2 cm
R
V
I   1 cm
X

UNEFFACED

DILATATION OF CERVIX

0   1   2   3   4   5   6   7   8   9   10   11   12

HOURS AFTER ADMISSION

F   160
E
T   150
A
L   140

130
H
E   120
A
R   110
T
100

FETAL HEART

LIQUOR

OXYTOCIN

ANALGESIA

Time of Delivery .... Method .... Duration ....

DURATION OF LABOUR

The duration of labour is recorded as the interval between Time of Admission and Time of Delivery. This equates with the number of hours a woman spends in the delivery unit before her baby is born. No allowance is made for time spent at home.

The duration of labour is expressed in this manner because: (i) mothers decide the time of admission; (ii) doctors and midwives assume their responsibility at that point; and (iii) accurate records demand precise information, which permits comparisons to be made.

The same procedure is followed when a woman is admitted to the delivery unit for induction because the pressures are identical, although the woman may not be in labour for much of the time, and sometimes not at all should induction fail and delivery be effected by caesarean section.

The duration of labour is effectively determined by the first stage. The second stage is very short by comparison. The third stage is not included.

GRAPH 2

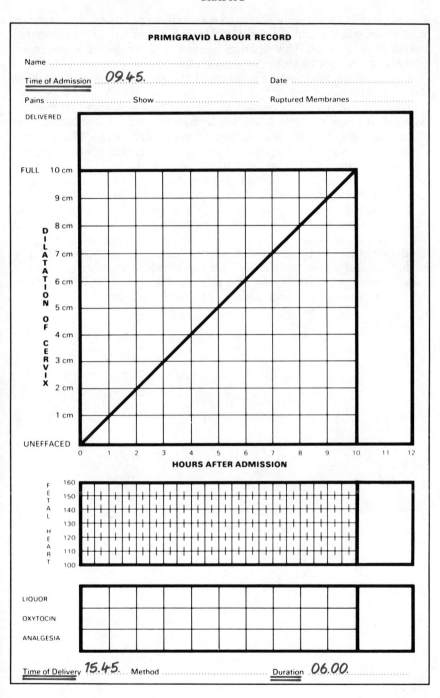

PRIMIGRAVID LABOUR RECORD

Name ....

Time of Admission ...09.45... .... Date ....

Pains .... Show .... Ruptured Membranes ....

DELIVERED

FULL   10 cm

9 cm

8 cm

D I L A T A T I O N   O F   C E R V I X   7 cm

6 cm

5 cm

4 cm

3 cm

2 cm

1 cm

UNEFFACED

0   1   2   3   4   5   6   7   8   9   10   11   12

HOURS AFTER ADMISSION

F E T A L   H E A R T   160 150 140 130 120 110 100

LIQUOR

OXYTOCIN

ANALGESIA

Time of Delivery *15.45.* Method .... Duration ...06.00.....................

DIAGNOSIS OF LABOUR

This is the most important item in the management of labour. All diagnoses must be prospective and a diagnosis of labour means a decision to commit a woman to delivery. This decision is made and the evidence placed on permanent record not later than one hour after admission.

Pain is an essential feature of labour, but a medical diagnosis of labour should not rest on pain alone.

Dilatation of the cervix constitutes the only proof of labour. Hence it is essential to know precisely what this term means and to understand that effacement must be completed before dilatation can begin. The problem arises when a woman admits herself with painful uterine contractions but without complete effacement, and therefore without dilatation. A 'show' or ruptured membranes, although not conclusive, is an invaluable aid to diagnosis in these circumstances, because both are objective in nature.

This particular case record represents a woman who admits herself to hospital because she believes herself to be in labour on the basis of painful uterine contractions and a 'show'. The cervix is not effaced completely, so there is no question of dilatation. A positive diagnosis is made, nevertheless, because painful uterine contractions are supported by objective evidence, in this case a 'show'. A similar decision is made when painful uterine contractions are supported by spontaneous rupture of membranes.

GRAPH 3

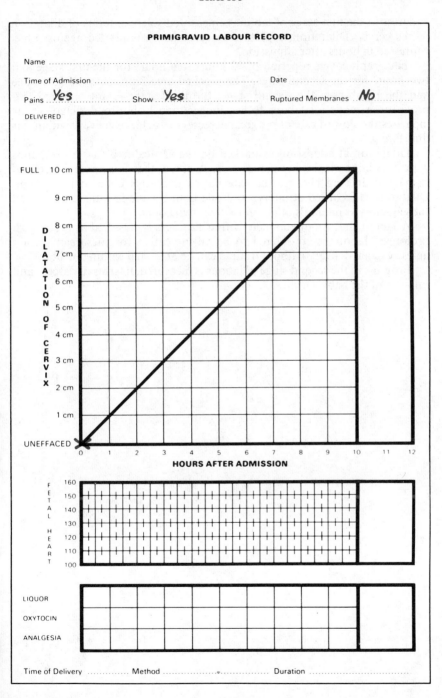

PRIMIGRAVID LABOUR RECORD

Name ....

Time of Admission .... Date ....

Pains .. *Yes* .... Show ... *Yes* .... Ruptured Membranes . *No* ....

DELIVERED

DILATATION OF CERVIX

FULL   10 cm

9 cm

8 cm

7 cm

6 cm

5 cm

4 cm

3 cm

2 cm

1 cm

UNEFFACED

0   1   2   3   4   5   6   7   8   9   10   11   12

HOURS AFTER ADMISSION

FETAL HEART

160
150
140
130
120
110
100

LIQUOR

OXYTOCIN

ANALGESIA

Time of Delivery .... Method .... Duration ....

PROGRESS IN LABOUR

Progress in the first stage of labour is measured solely in terms of dilatation of the cervix. Dilatation, expressed in centimetres, is plotted against time, expressed in hours after admission.

The graph covers a period of 12 hours: ten hours for the first stage and two hours for the second stage. The blocked area represents the first stage and the blank area the second stage; the third stage is not included. No provision is made for labour to last longer than 12 hours. A diagonal line indicates the slowest rate of progress necessary to achieve delivery within this time limit.

Dilatation at admission is marked on the vertical axis that corresponds with zero hour on the horizontal axis. A cervix that is completely effaced is marked at 1 cm because the external os is always open to this extent. Dilatation is recorded at intervals of one hour for the first three hours and subsequently at intervals of not more than two hours.

A labour that is not complete within 12 hours is classified as prolonged. Prolonged labour is considered to be an indication for caesarean section unless vaginal delivery without trauma can be predicted within one hour.

Progress in the second stage of labour is measured in terms of descent and rotation of the baby's head.

GRAPH 4

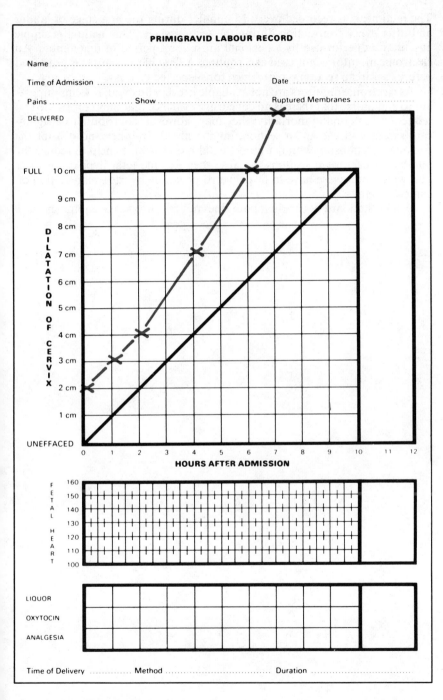

FETAL HEART

The fetal heart is recorded every 15 minutes during the first stage of labour and after every contraction during the second stage. The method is simple auscultation performed by a personal nurse for a period of one minute. An electronic monitor is not used as a routine. A fetal blood sample is examined before caesarean section is performed for suspected distress.

As electronic monitors are not available in every hospital, it seems important to emphasize that there is no conclusive evidence that they contribute to a reduction in perinatal mortality; they may, however, contribute to a significant increase in caesarean section, immobilize the mother and disrupt the personal relationship with her nurse. Fetal blood samples help to reduce the number of caesarean sections, because they exclude fetal hypoxia in cases that would otherwise have to be delivered promptly by caesarean section on clinical grounds.

A high standard of care in labour does not require special equipment.

GRAPH 5

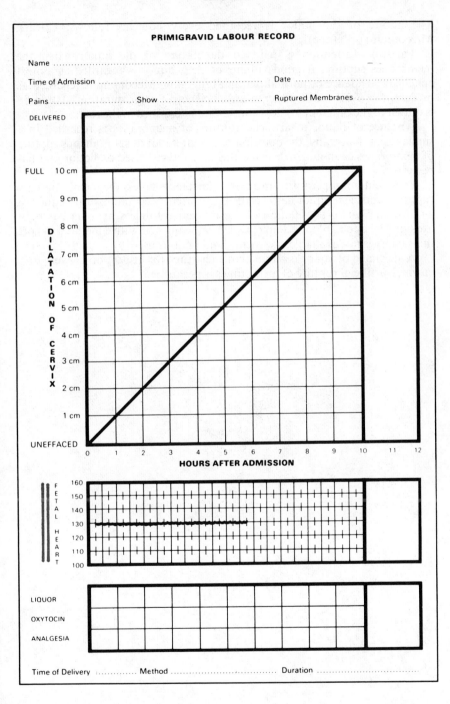

PRIMIGRAVID LABOUR RECORD

Name .... — ‾

Time of Admission .... Date ....

Pains .... Show .... Ruptured Membranes ....

DELIVERED

FULL 10 cm

9 cm

8 cm

D I L A T A T I O N   O F   C E R V I X

7 cm

6 cm

5 cm

4 cm

3 cm

2 cm

1 cm

UNEFFACED

0   1   2   3   4   5   6   7   8   9   10   11   12

HOURS AFTER ADMISSION

F E T A L   H E A R T

160
150
140
130
120
110
100

LIQUOR

OXYTOCIN

ANALGESIA

Time of Delivery .... Method .... Duration ....

LIQUOR

The nature of the liquor is recorded every hour as follows: C(lear), M(econium) or N(one).

Particular attention is paid to the nature of the liquor when the membranes rupture. A good volume of clear liquor is regarded as almost conclusive evidence of normal placental function. Meconium is regarded as presumptive evidence of placental insufficiency of some duration. Attention is drawn to the different grades of meconium described in the text.

Absence of liquor at artificial rupture of membranes is regarded in a similar light. Naturally, the question of absent liquor at spontaneous rupture of membranes cannot arise because this diagnosis is based on liquor that has been seen.

Oxytocin is not permitted in any circumstances unless the membranes are ruptured and clear liquor has been demonstrated. Meconium, or no liquor, is an absolute bar to stimulation of uterine activity unless hypoxia has been excluded by a fetal blood sample, which is the only definitive method. Where this facility is not available, oxytocin should not be used.

A specimen of liquor is retained in a test-tube for inspection in every case in which artificial rupture of membranes is performed.

GRAPH 6

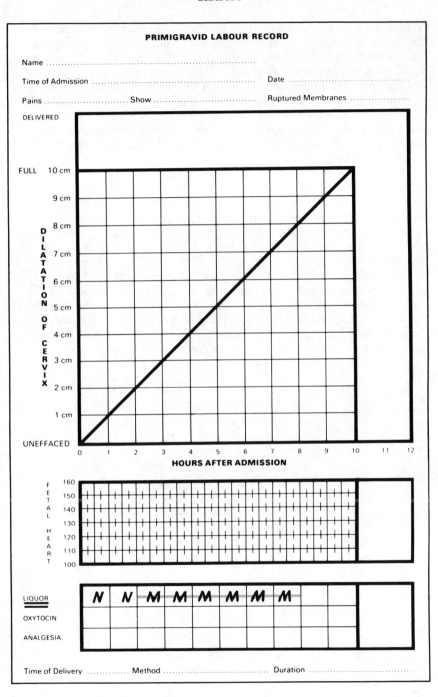

PRIMIGRAVID LABOUR RECORD

Name ....

Time of Admission ....   Date ....

Pains .... Show ....   Ruptured Membranes ....

DELIVERED

Dilatation of cervix (vertical axis):
FULL — 10 cm
9 cm
8 cm
7 cm
6 cm
5 cm
4 cm
3 cm
2 cm
1 cm
UNEFFACED

HOURS AFTER ADMISSION (0 to 12)

FETAL HEART:
160
150
140
130
120
110
100

LIQUOR   N N M M M M M M

OXYTOCIN

ANALGESIA

Time of Delivery .... Method .... Duration ....

128

OXYTOCIN

Whenever oxytocin is used—to induce or to accelerate—it is recorded in the space appropriate to Hours after Admission, which corresponds with Dilatation of Cervix on the same timescale. Oxytocin to induce begins at zero hour, whereas oxytocin to accelerate begins after an interval.

A solution of 10 units of oxytocin in 1 litre of 5% dextrose is used in all circumstances. The rate of infusion begins at 10 drops and increases every 15 minutes to a maximum of 60 drops per minute. Neither the concentration nor the rate nor the volume is exceeded. No special equipment is used. A simple gravity feed is regulated by the personal nurse, who cares for every woman in labour.

The number of contractions during each period of 15 minutes is recorded in serial fashion on the reverse side of the chart. The aim is five contractions in each period of 15 minutes. Above this number the rate of infusion tends to increase the force rather than the frequency of contractions, but should the frequency exceed seven contractions, the rate of infusion is adjusted accordingly. Oxytocin is not permitted unless the membranes are ruptured and clear liquor is seen.

Oxytocin is an extraordinarily effective drug when used to accelerate labour. Its effective use is often inhibited by fear of cephalopelvic disproportion, rupture of the uterus and trauma to the child. There is no foundation for any of these fears in primigravidae. A fundamental distinction must be made between primigravidae and multigravidae in respect of oxytocin. Oxytocin must be regarded as a dangerous drug in multigravidae.

Time	Rate	Contractions
12.00	10	1, 2
12.15	20	3, 4, 5
12.30	30	6, 7, 8
12.45	40	9, 10, 11
13.00	50	12, 13, 14, 15
13.15	60	16, 17, 18, 19, 20

GRAPH 7

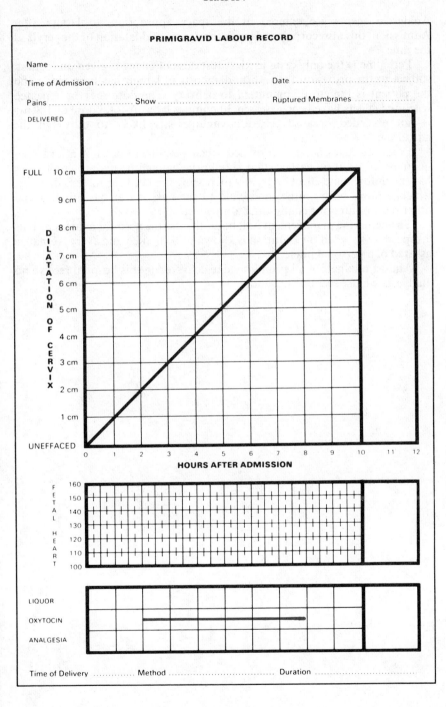

PRIMIGRAVID LABOUR RECORD

Name ....

Time of Admission .... Date ....

Pains .... Show .... Ruptured Membranes ....

DELIVERED

DILATATION OF CERVIX

FULL 10 cm
9 cm
8 cm
7 cm
6 cm
5 cm
4 cm
3 cm
2 cm
1 cm
UNEFFACED

0 1 2 3 4 5 6 7 8 9 10 11 12

HOURS AFTER ADMISSION

FETAL HEART

160
150
140
130
120
110
100

LIQUOR

OXYTOCIN

ANALGESIA

Time of Delivery .... Method .... Duration ....

130

ANALGESIA

Analgesic agents are entered in the space appropriate to Hours after Admission; this also corresponds with the degree of dilatation of the cervix at the time.

Pethidine is the only drug used. A test dose of 50 mg is given on request, subject to the provision that a firm diagnosis of labour has been made and the patient is therefore committed to delivery. The dose may be repeated when the effects have been assessed 30 minutes later. A total dose of 100 mg is not exceeded because the disadvantages are likely to outweigh the advantages.

Epidural anaesthesia is provided when pethidine does not afford adequate relief, or at an earlier stage should the woman be unduly upset. This has the unfortunate effect of greatly increasing the need for forceps delivery, which exposes both mother and child to the risk of trauma. For this and other reasons no prior commitments are given.

The better the management of labour, the less the need for analgesia. This is especially so when the duration is known to be limited and every woman is assured of a personal nurse.

Almost one-half of all primigravidae delivered in this hospital receive no analgesia whatsoever during labour.

GRAPH 8

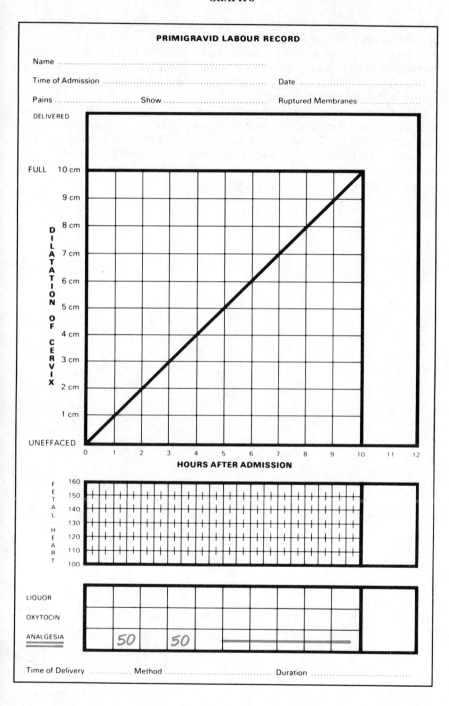

PRIMIGRAVID LABOUR RECORD

Name ....

Time of Admission .... Date ....

Pains .... Show .... Ruptured Membranes ....

DELIVERED

FULL   10 cm

9 cm

8 cm

D
I 7 cm
L
A
T 6 cm
A
T
I 5 cm
O
N

O 4 cm
F

C 3 cm
E
R
V 2 cm
I
X

1 cm

UNEFFACED

0   1   2   3   4   5   6   7   8   9   10   11   12

HOURS AFTER ADMISSION

F   160
E
T   150
A
L   140

130
H
E   120
A
R   110
T
100

LIQUOR

OXYTOCIN

ANALGESIA   50   50

Time of Delivery .... Method .... Duration ....

METHOD OF DELIVERY AND ADDITIONAL ITEMS

Method of delivery is recorded as: Spontaneous, Forceps or Caesarean Section, as the case may be.

The only additional items permitted are: spontaneous rupture of membranes (SRM), artificial rupture of membranes (ARM), fetal blood sample (FBS), and electronic fetal monitor (EFM). These are entered directly on the graph, in the appropriate place.

The temptation to include more and more information simply because it is available or to ensure that nothing conceivable is omitted that might appear desirable for the purpose of study at some future date must be resisted as contrary to the whole purpose of the exercise, which is the instant visual impact of a small number of essential items. Retrospective studies of this nature are rarely of value in any event.

GRAPH 9

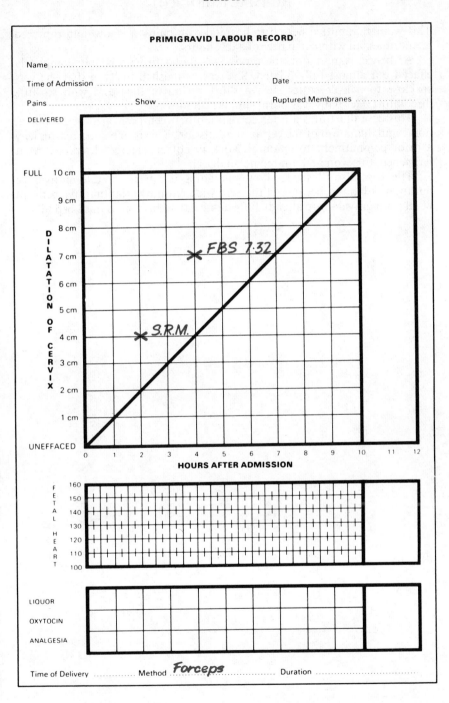

PRIMIGRAVID LABOUR RECORD

Name ....

Time of Admission .... Date ....

Pains .... Show .... Ruptured Membranes ....

DELIVERED

FULL   10 cm

9 cm

8 cm

D
I
L
A   7 cm   ✗ *FBS 7·32*
T
A
T   6 cm
I
O
N   5 cm

O
F   4 cm   ✗ *S.R.M.*

C
E   3 cm
R
V
I   2 cm
X

1 cm

UNEFFACED
          0   1   2   3   4   5   6   7   8   9   10   11   12
                    HOURS AFTER ADMISSION

F   160
E   150
T
A   140
L
    130
H
E   120
A
R   110
T   100

LIQUOR

OXYTOCIN

ANALGESIA

Time of Delivery .... Method *Forceps* .... Duration ....

NORMAL LABOUR (1)

This woman admitted herself to hospital with pains, a 'show' and ruptured membranes, all within a matter of a few hours.

At pelvic examination the cervix was found to be not only completely effaced but almost fully dilated. She was astonished to learn that she was so close to delivery after such a short period of time and with so little discomfort. Her baby was born within the hour.

This case illustrates a poor correlation between time spent in labour at home and dilatation of the cervix at admission. This is one good reason why a prior commitment to epidural block is not considered desirable. As it happened, this woman required no analgesia.

This case also illustrates how misleading it can be to state an average duration of labour, because of the very wide natural variation. Five per cent of all primigravidae are already fully dilated at admission to this hospital.

GRAPH 10

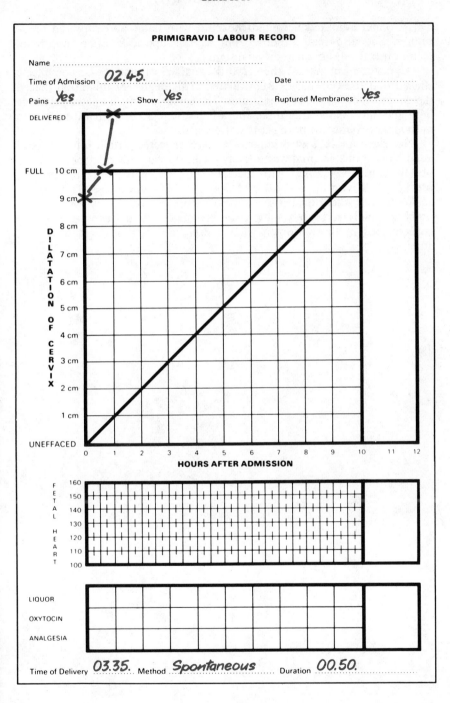

PRIMIGRAVID LABOUR RECORD

Name ....

Time of Admission ..*02.45.*..................... Date ....

Pains ..*Yes*.............. Show ..*Yes*.................... Ruptured Membranes ..*Yes*..........

DELIVERED

FULL 10 cm

9 cm

8 cm

7 cm

6 cm

5 cm

4 cm

3 cm

2 cm

1 cm

UNEFFACED

DILATATION OF CERVIX

0 1 2 3 4 5 6 7 8 9 10 11 12

HOURS AFTER ADMISSION

FETAL HEART

160
150
140
130
120
110
100

LIQUOR

OXYTOCIN

ANALGESIA

Time of Delivery ..*03.35.*.. Method ..*Spontaneous*........... Duration ..*00.50.*..............

NORMAL LABOUR (2)

This woman admitted herself to hospital with pains and ruptured membranes. She also had a 'show', but as this appeared after rupture of membranes it was not an additional sign.

At pelvic examination the cervical canal was found to be completely effaced and the external os 3 cm dilated. This degree of dilatation placed the diagnosis of labour beyond doubt. The cervix was 5 cm dilated after one hour and fully dilated after three-and-a-half hours. Soon she felt the desire to push and her baby was born shortly afterwards.

No less than 40% of primigravidae are delivered within four hours of admission to this hospital without any medical treatment whatsoever. Some obstetricians not familiar with the facts in this regard speak in terms of precipitate delivery in the context of labour of this duration (see Table 8).

Women in whom the cervix is 2 cm or more dilated at admission tend to proceed rapidly and rarely suffer from prolonged labour. The problems are concentrated in those women whose cervix is less than 2 cm dilated at admission.

GRAPH 11

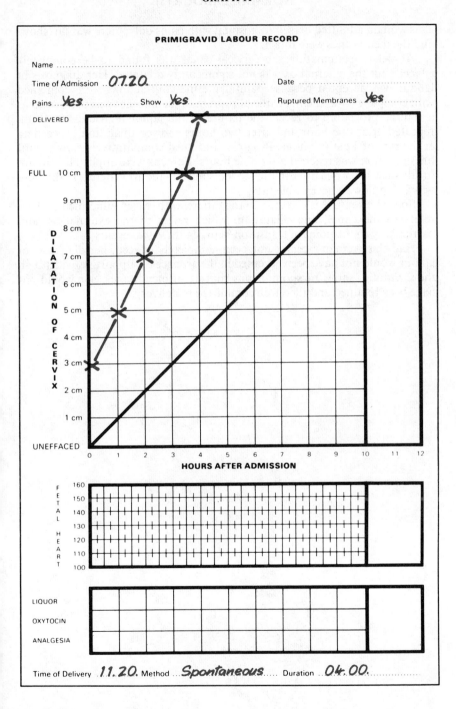

PRIMIGRAVID LABOUR RECORD

Name ....

Time of Admission .. *07.20.* .... Date ....

Pains .. *Yes* .... Show .. *Yes* .... Ruptured Membranes .. *Yes* ....

DELIVERED

FULL 10 cm

D
I
L
A
T
A
T
I
O
N

O
F

C
E
R
V
I
X

9 cm

8 cm

7 cm

6 cm

5 cm

4 cm

3 cm

2 cm

1 cm

UNEFFACED

0   1   2   3   4   5   6   7   8   9   10   11   12

HOURS AFTER ADMISSION

F E T A L   H E A R T
160
150
140
130
120
110
100

LIQUOR

OXYTOCIN

ANALGESIA

Time of Delivery *11.20.* Method *Spontaneous* Duration *04.00.*

NORMAL LABOUR (3)

This woman admitted herself to hospital with pains only; there was no 'show' and the membranes were intact.

At pelvic examination the cervical canal was found to be completely effaced, but the external os was not significantly dilatated. Her diagnosis of labour was accepted because painful uterine contractions were combined with complete effacement. Artificial rupture of membranes was performed as a routine procedure to reveal the nature of the liquor. Pelvic examination repeated after one hour and after two hours showed dilatation proceeding at the rate of 1 cm per hour. Progress continued comparatively slowly until full dilatation was reached after nine hours. Forceps were applied for failure to advance, after one hour in the second stage of labour. Progress in this case was at the slowest acceptable rate.

Special attention is directed to the difference between effacement, which refers to the canal, and dilatation, which refers to the external os, and particularly to the point of transition between these two events.

Had this woman's cervix not been completely effaced, her diagnosis of labour would not have been accepted in the absence of supportive evidence in the form of a 'show' or spontaneous rupture of membranes. She would not have been retained and therefore committed to delivery.

GRAPH 12

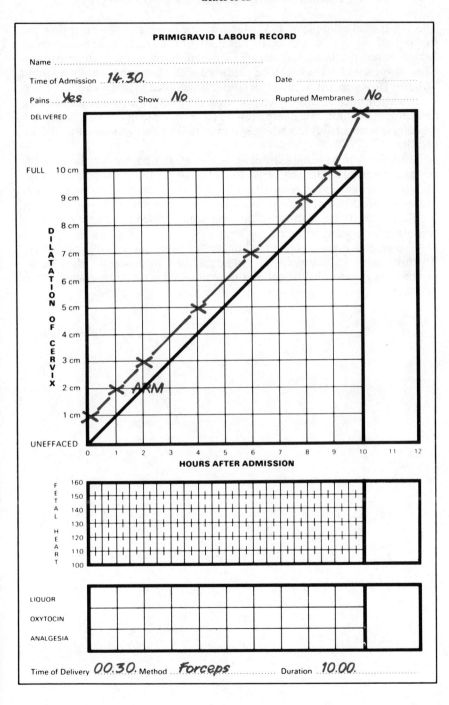

PRIMIGRAVID LABOUR RECORD

Name ....

Time of Admission ..*14.30.*.. Date ....

Pains ...*Yes*................. Show ...*No*......................... Ruptured Membranes ..*No*.............

DELIVERED

FULL   10 cm

9 cm

8 cm

D I L A T A T I O N   O F   C E R V I X   7 cm

6 cm

5 cm

4 cm

3 cm

2 cm   *ARM*

1 cm

UNEFFACED

0 1 2 3 4 5 6 7 8 9 10 11 12

HOURS AFTER ADMISSION

F E T A L   H E A R T

160
150
140
130
120
110
100

LIQUOR

OXYTOCIN

ANALGESIA

Time of Delivery *00.30.* Method *Forceps* .... Duration *10.00.*......................

ABNORMAL LABOUR: SLOW PROGRESS (1)

This is a typical example of a hypothetical case in which progress is slow but steady and the cervix is close to full dilatation after 12 hours. Caesarean section is not performed on a rule of thumb basis in these circumstances when safe vaginal delivery can be predicted with reasonable certainty within an hour. However, the duration of labour is recorded as abnormal.

A woman such as this is likely to show evidence of incipient dehydration and ketosis; her morale is almost sure to have begun to deteriorate badly and on achievement of full dilatation she may well be too exhausted to deliver herself.

She is likely to have unpleasant memories of childbirth if only because she will have received a relatively large dose of analgesic drugs to compensate for the length of her labour; her baby is more likely to have a low Apgar score and to require admission to a special care unit for 24 hours.

These undesirable features could have been avoided were action taken to accelerate progress at six hours.

This case record should be read in conjunction with the two that follow. All three cases are examples of primary failure to progress, which is invariably the result of inefficient uterine action and is therefore responsive to oxytocin.

GRAPH 13

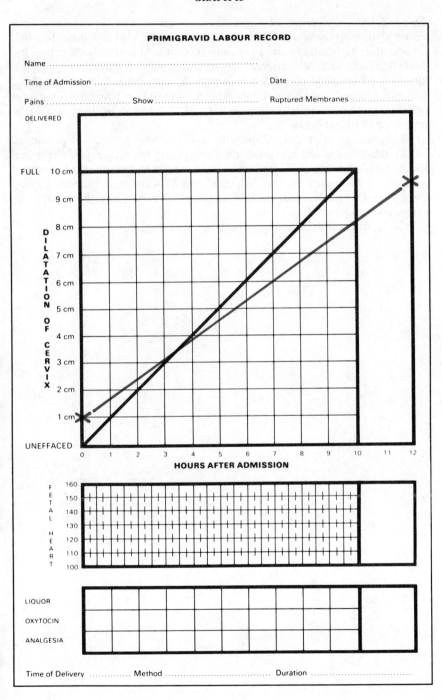

PRIMIGRAVID LABOUR RECORD

Name ....

Time of Admission .... Date ....

Pains .... Show .... Ruptured Membranes ....

DELIVERED

FULL

DILATATION OF CERVIX

10 cm
9 cm
8 cm
7 cm
6 cm
5 cm
4 cm
3 cm
2 cm
1 cm

UNEFFACED

0 1 2 3 4 5 6 7 8 9 10 11 12

HOURS AFTER ADMISSION

FETAL HEART

160
150
140
130
120
110
100

LIQUOR

OXYTOCIN

ANALGESIA

Time of Delivery .... Method .... Duration ....

ABNORMAL LABOUR: SLOW PROGRESS (2)

This is a second example of a hypothetical case in which progress is even slower than in the previous instance, so that the cervix is little more than half dilated after 12 hours. In these circumstances it is abundantly clear that full dilatation will not be achieved for several hours. Furthermore, there is always the likelihood of a difficult forceps delivery because the baby's head may not descend and rotate. This particular situation is fraught with serious risk of trauma to both mother and child. Caesarean section should be performed without delay.

A woman such as this is bound to suffer from the effects of prolonged labour described in the previous case and to carry the memory of the ordeal for the rest of her life. In addition, she has a caesarean section scar to contend with in any future pregnancy. A special note of warning is sounded against the misuse of epidural anaesthesia to permit the duration of labour to be extended even longer.

Corrective action should have been taken at three hours.

GRAPH 14

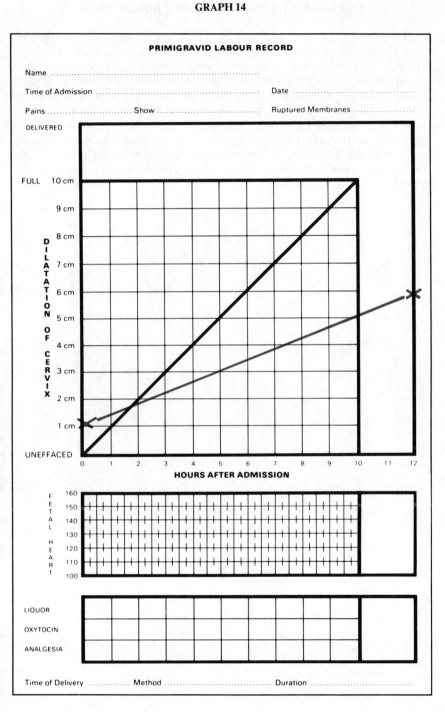

PRIMIGRAVID LABOUR RECORD

Name ....

Time of Admission .... Date ....

Pains .... Show .... Ruptured Membranes ....

DELIVERED

FULL 10 cm

9 cm

8 cm

DILATATION OF CERVIX

7 cm

6 cm

5 cm

4 cm

3 cm

2 cm

1 cm

UNEFFACED

0 1 2 3 4 5 6 7 8 9 10 11 12

HOURS AFTER ADMISSION

FETAL HEART

160
150
140
130
120
110
100

LIQUOR

OXYTOCIN

ANALGESIA

Time of Delivery .... Method .... Duration ....

ABNORMAL LABOUR: SLOW PROGRESS (3)

This is a third example of a hypothetical case in which progress is negligible from the beginning and the cervix is less than half dilatated after 12 hours. There should be no hesitation whatsoever in deciding treatment in these circumstances, because there is no telling when, if ever, the cervix will reach full dilatation. A woman such as this is set on a course that is likely to end in disaster. Caesarean section should be performed without further delay.

Progress should have been accelerated as early as two hours after admission in this case. Early detection of slow progress depends on regular pelvic examination during the first three hours. Abnormal patterns of labour are tacitly accepted when pelvic examination is performed at intervals of four hours.

GRAPH 15

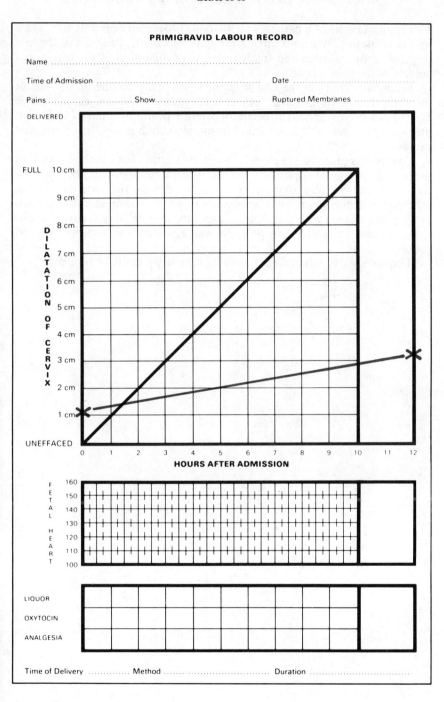

PRIMIGRAVID LABOUR RECORD

Name ....

Time of Admission .... Date ....

Pains .... Show .... Ruptured Membranes ....

DELIVERED

FULL   10 cm

9 cm

8 cm

D
I
L   7 cm
A
T   6 cm
A
T   5 cm
I
O   4 cm
N

O   3 cm
F

C   2 cm
E
R   1 cm
V
I
X

UNEFFACED

0   1   2   3   4   5   6   7   8   9   10   11   12

HOURS AFTER ADMISSION

F   160
E
T   150
A
L   140

130
H
E   120
A
R   110
T
100

LIQUOR

OXYTOCIN

ANALGESIA

Time of Delivery .... Method .... Duration ....

ABNORMAL LABOUR: SECONDARY ARREST (1)

This is an example of a case in which labour proceeded normally until close on full dilatation, when no further progress was made. Progress in the first stage of labour is measured solely in terms of dilatation of the cervix, not descent of the baby's head.

Secondary arrest in the first stage of labour may be due to any one of the three causes of dystocia, but is more characteristic of cephalopelvic disproportion—or persistent occipitoposterior position—than of inefficient uterine action. Nevertheless, inefficient uterine action is still the commonest cause.

Oxytocin is given to ensure efficient uterine action for a limited period of time, without fear of rupture of the uterus (in a primigravida) or injury to the child. In this way oxytocin is used to identify the case of genuine cephalopelvic disproportion. Caesarean section is performed unless normal progress is resumed within an hour. As spontaneous delivery occurred in this case, the secondary arrest in progress was attributed to inefficient uterine action.

The outcome in this and the following case might easily be reversed.

GRAPH 16

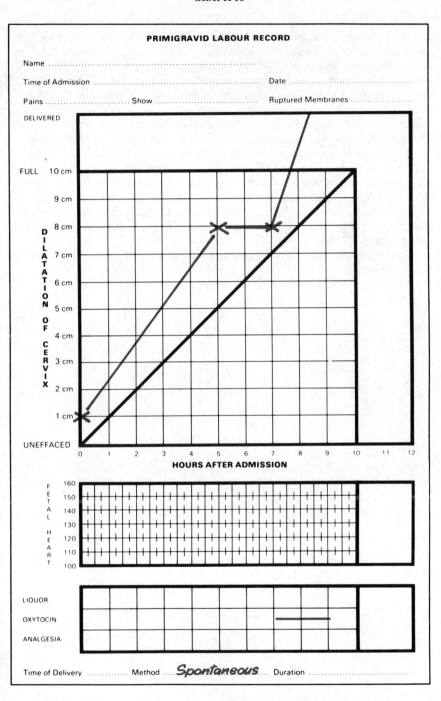

PRIMIGRAVID LABOUR RECORD

Name ....

Time of Admission ....   Date ....

Pains ....   Show ....   Ruptured Membranes ....

DELIVERED

FULL   10 cm

9 cm

8 cm

D 7 cm
I
L 6 cm
A
T 5 cm
A
T 4 cm
I
O 3 cm
N
   2 cm
O
F 1 cm

C
E UNEFFACED
R   0   1   2   3   4   5   6   7   8   9   10   11   12
V
I   **HOURS AFTER ADMISSION**
X

F 160
E 150
T
A 140
L
   130
H
E 120
A 110
R
T 100

LIQUOR

OXYTOCIN

ANALGESIA

Time of Delivery ....   Method .... *Spontaneous* ...   Duration ....

ABNORMAL LABOUR: SECONDARY ARREST (2)

This is an example similar in all respects to the previous case, except that labour proceeded normally until full dilatation, after which no further progress was made. Progress in the second stage of labour is measured solely in terms of descent and rotation of the baby's head.

Secondary arrest in the second stage, which presents as failure of the head to descend to the level of the pelvic floor, may likewise be due to any one of the three causes of dystocia, but again is more characteristic of cephalopelvic disproportion—or persistent occipitoposterior position—than of inefficient uterine action, although the latter is still the most likely cause.

The method of treatment is the same as in the first stage of labour. Oxytocin is given to ensure efficient uterine action for a limited period of time. Caesarean section is performed unless the head has reached the pelvic floor within an hour. The one option not available is forcible extraction through the undilatated vagina, with the head high and in the transverse diameter of the pelvis. This has been referred to in the text as phase one of the second stage of labour.

Secondary arrest in phase two of the second stage of labour is treated by low forceps.

The final diagnosis in this case was cephalopelvic disproportion.

GRAPH 17

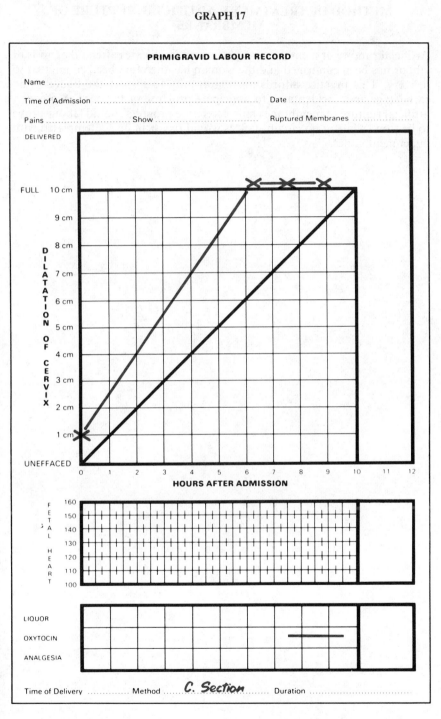

PRIMIGRAVID LABOUR RECORD

Name ....

Time of Admission .... Date ....

Pains .... Show .... Ruptured Membranes ....

DELIVERED

FULL   10 cm

9 cm

8 cm

DILATATION OF CERVIX

7 cm

6 cm

5 cm

4 cm

3 cm

2 cm

1 cm

UNEFFACED

0   1   2   3   4   5   6   7   8   9   10   11   12

HOURS AFTER ADMISSION

FETAL HEART

160
150
140
130
120
110
100

LIQUOR

OXYTOCIN

ANALGESIA

Time of Delivery .... Method .... *C. Section* .... Duration ....

METHOD OF TREATMENT: ARTIFICIAL RUPTURE OF MEMBRANES

Artificial rupture of membranes is performed in all cases after a diagnosis of labour has been confirmed and the woman has therefore been committed to delivery. This practice affords an opportunity to inspect the liquor at an early stage and, incidentally, to anticipate prolapse of the cord. Moreover, artificial rupture of membranes may accelerate progress should labour prove to be slow, while in no circumstances would oxytocin be contemplated with intact membranes.

GRAPH 18

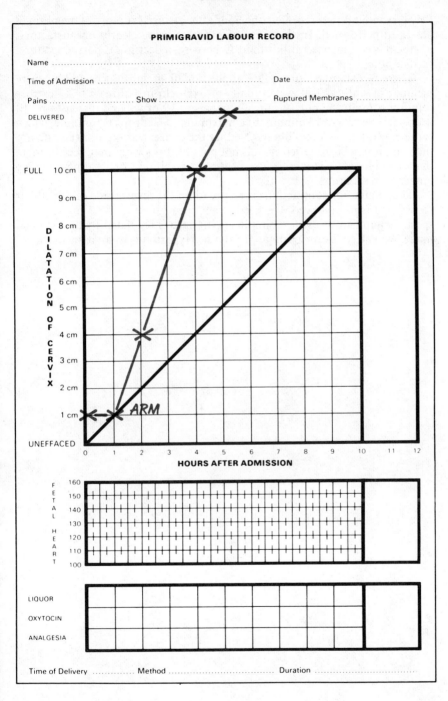

PRIMIGRAVID LABOUR RECORD

Name ....

Time of Admission .... Date ....

Pains .... Show .... Ruptured Membranes ....

DELIVERED

FULL 10 cm

9 cm

8 cm

D I L A T A T I O N   O F   C E R V I X

7 cm

6 cm

5 cm

4 cm

3 cm

2 cm

1 cm ARM

UNEFFACED

0 1 2 3 4 5 6 7 8 9 10 11 12

HOURS AFTER ADMISSION

FETAL HEART

160
150
140
130
120
110
100

LIQUOR

OXYTOCIN

ANALGESIA

Time of Delivery .... Method .... Duration ....

METHOD OF TREATMENT: OXYTOCIN INFUSION (1)

Pelvic examination is repeated one hour after artificial rupture of membranes has been performed. In the event of progress being clearly unsatisfactory, oxytocin is commenced at this time. Otherwise, a decision is postponed for a further hour.

There is a standard procedure applied in all circumstances and by every member of staff, as follows: 10 units of oxytocin in 1 litre of 5% dextrose solution is used; the rate of infusion begins at 10 drops and increases by 10 drops at intervals of 15 minutes to a maximum of 60 drops per minute, which is the equivalent of 40 milliunits. Neither the concentration, nor the rate nor the volume can be exceeded, so it is not possible for a woman to receive more than 10 units of oxytocin, 1 litre of dextrose solution or treatment lasting longer than six hours.

The number of contractions is recorded on the reverse side of the labour record and is not allowed to exceed seven in each period of 15 minutes. No special equipment is used. A simple gravity feed is regulated by the personal nurse, who attends every woman in labour. Hypertonus is not a problem.

GRAPH 19

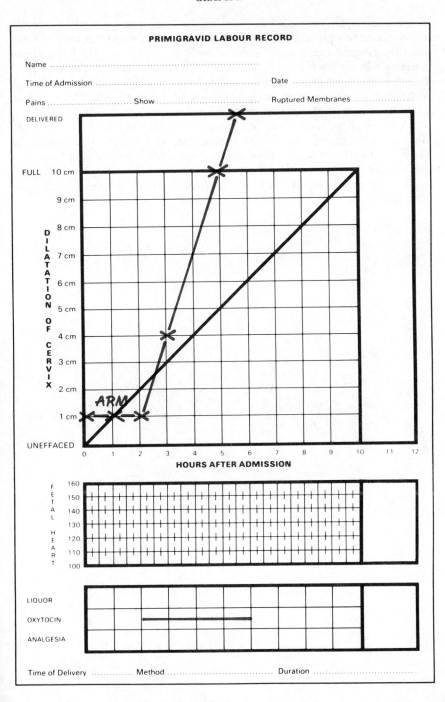

PRIMIGRAVID LABOUR RECORD

Name ....

Time of Admission .... Date ....

Pains .... Show .... Ruptured Membranes ....

DELIVERED

FULL   10 cm

9 cm

8 cm

**D
I
L
A
T
A
T
I
O
N

O
F

C
E
R
V
I
X**

7 cm

6 cm

5 cm

4 cm

3 cm

2 cm

ARM

1 cm

UNEFFACED

0   1   2   3   4   5   6   7   8   9   10   11   12

HOURS AFTER ADMISSION

**F
E
T
A
L

H
E
A
R
T**

160
150
140
130
120
110
100

LIQUOR

OXYTOCIN

ANALGESIA

Time of Delivery .... Method .... Duration ....

METHOD OF TREATMENT: OXYTOCIN INFUSION (2)

There is a relatively small but none the less important group of cases in which the cervix proceeds to full dilatation within a normal period of time, but then progress ceases early in the second stage of labour. The baby's head remains high in the transverse position. The mother has no desire to push because there is no pressure on her pelvic floor. The obstetrician is faced with a choice between caesarean section and difficult rotation and extraction. Too often he chooses the latter course simply because the cervix is fully dilated.

A standard oxytocin infusion introduced at this juncture more often than not results in resumption of normal progress, with descent and rotation of head. A difficult and potentially dangerous situation is converted into an easy forceps, if not spontaneous, delivery.

Thus oxytocin can also be an invaluable aid to management of the second stage of labour.

GRAPH 20

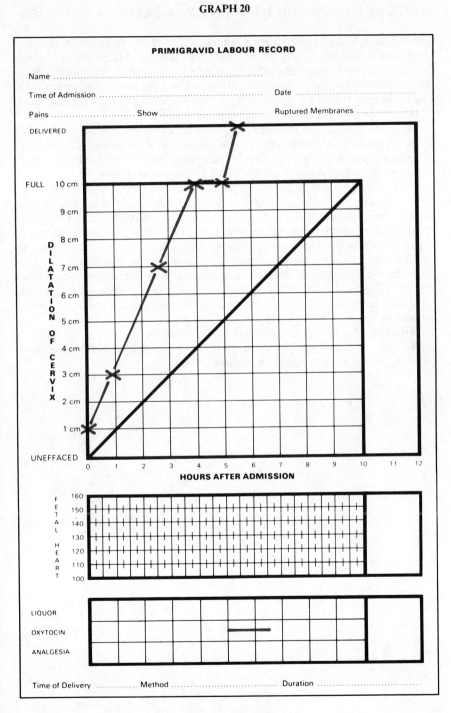

PRIMIGRAVID LABOUR RECORD

Name ....

Time of Admission .... Date ....

Pains .... Show .... Ruptured Membranes ....

DELIVERED

FULL   10 cm

D
I   9 cm
L
A   8 cm
T
A   7 cm
T
I   6 cm
O
N   5 cm
O
F   4 cm
C   3 cm
E
R   2 cm
V
I   1 cm
X
UNEFFACED

0   1   2   3   4   5   6   7   8   9   10   11   12

HOURS AFTER ADMISSION

F   160
E   150
T   140
A
L   130
H   120
E   110
A
R   100
T

LIQUOR

OXYTOCIN

ANALGESIA

Time of Delivery .... Method .... Duration ....

FAILURE TO RESPOND TO TREATMENT: ERROR IN DIAGNOSIS

Far the most likely explanation of failure to respond to treatment is an error in diagnosis. Expressed in simple terms, this means that the woman is not in labour. The error arises when diagnosis is based on subjective evidence only. The uterus in labour is so uniformly sensitive that oxytocin is an almost infallible test; this is assuredly not so with the uterus not in labour, as all familiar with the problems of induction well know.

When oxytocin fails to accelerate, treatment is discontinued—preferably after 0.5 litres, which takes about three hours—until the case is reviewed and a formal decision taken as to whether to attempt to retrieve the error and so return to the original position or proceed to caesarean section.

The final decision depends largely on the emotional condition of the mother at the time. When the first option is chosen she is removed from the delivery unit, hopefully to return in labour within a matter of hours. In either event, it is considered a matter of great importance that this most frequent of errors in labour management should be duly recognized and that caesarean section performed in these circumstances should not be attributed to a false indication, most likely dystocia—caused by inefficient uterine action, persistent occipitoposterior position or cephalopelvic disproportion—when a state of labour never existed. The situation is analogous to failed induction, where similar misunderstandings arise.

Incidentally, this pattern of primary failure of the cervix to dilate is never due to cephalopelvic disproportion or persistent occipitoposterior position, but always to inefficient uterine action.

GRAPH 21

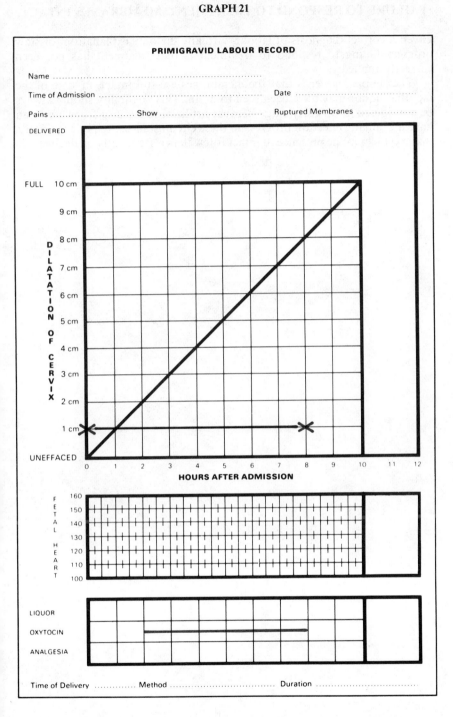

PRIMIGRAVID LABOUR RECORD

Name ....

Time of Admission .... Date ....

Pains .... Show .... Ruptured Membranes ....

DELIVERED

FULL 10 cm

9 cm

8 cm

D I L A T A T I O N   O F   C E R V I X

7 cm

6 cm

5 cm

4 cm

3 cm

2 cm

1 cm

UNEFFACED

0 1 2 3 4 5 6 7 8 9 10 11 12

HOURS AFTER ADMISSION

F E T A L   H E A R T

160
150
140
130
120
110
100

LIQUOR

OXYTOCIN

ANALGESIA

Time of Delivery .... Method .... Duration ....

FAILURE TO RESPOND TO TREATMENT: MEMBRANES INTACT

Given a correct diagnosis of labour, virtually the only explanation for slow progress failing to respond to treatment is that treatment has not been correctly applied.

The simple answer is that the membranes are still intact, in spite of the fact that liquor may have been seen to drain. This possibility should always be considered at an early stage because artificial rupture of forewaters can have a dramatic effect on progress in these circumstances. Experience shows that oxytocin in the presence of intact forewaters is frequently ineffective.

GRAPH 22

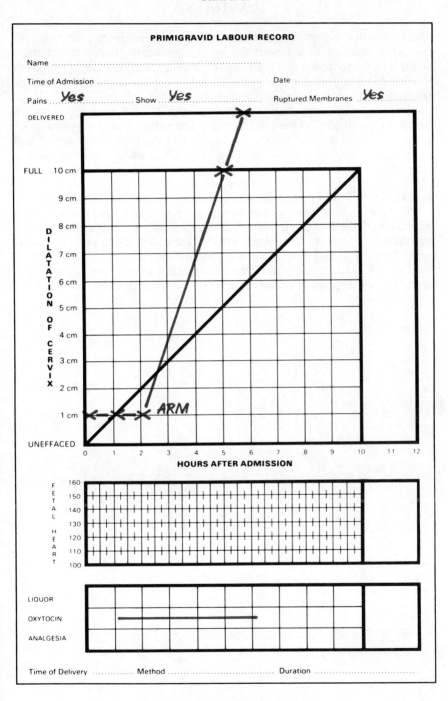

FAILURE TO RESPOND TO TREATMENT: HESITANT USE OF OXYTOCIN

Given both that a woman is in labour and that her membranes are ruptured, the explanation of slow labour failing to respond to treatment is almost surely that oxytocin has not been used in the prescribed manner. The reason for this is to be found in the sensitive area of interpersonal relationships between members of the medical and nursing staff.

The sister in charge of the delivery unit is sure to begin with an ambivalent attitude, because she has been trained to regard oxytocin as an extremely dangerous substance associated with rupture of the uterus and trauma to the child. Naturally, she does not wish to accept the responsibility unless the most explicit assurances are given at the highest level. As this is seldom the case in practice, treatment comes to nought, while obstetricians wonder how it is that similar measures can prove successful elsewhere.

Mutual confidence between nurses and doctors, and indeed mothers, is an essential ingredient of good labour management, but it needs to be carefully nurtured. The alternative is a high reported incidence of uterine hypertonus, with fetal distress and cephalopelvic disproportion.

This pattern of dilatation of the cervix is not in any way suggestive of cephalopelvic disproportion, or of persistent occipitoposterior position.

GRAPH 23

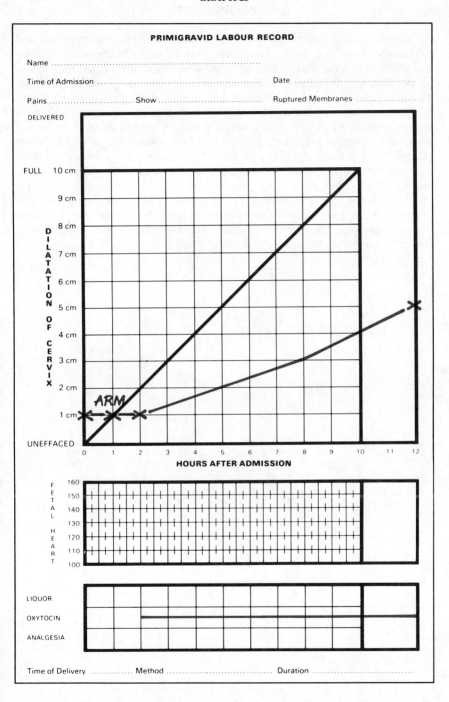

FAILURE TO RESPOND TO TREATMENT: CEPHALOPELVIC DISPROPORTION

Assuming the diagnosis of labour to be correct, the membranes ruptured and oxytocin to have been used in the prescribed manner, there remain but two reasons why labour may continue to be slow; these are cephalopelvic disproportion, and its clinical analogue, persistent occipitoposterior position. These two can be considered together because the clinical picture is identical.

The characteristic feature of cephalopelvic disproportion, and persistent occipitoposterior position, is failure of the baby's head to descend in spite of progressive dilatation of the cervix, which bears witness to efficient uterine action. Sometimes this failure of the head to descend is associated with secondary arrest in dilatation of the cervix late in the first stage of labour, and at other times the cervix proceeds to full dilatation with the same outcome. Even in these circumstances a diagnosis of cephalopelvic disproportion, or persistent occipitoposterior position can seldom be made without oxytocin to ensure efficient uterine action. X-ray pelvimetry contributes nothing to the solution of this essentially clinical problem.

GRAPH 24

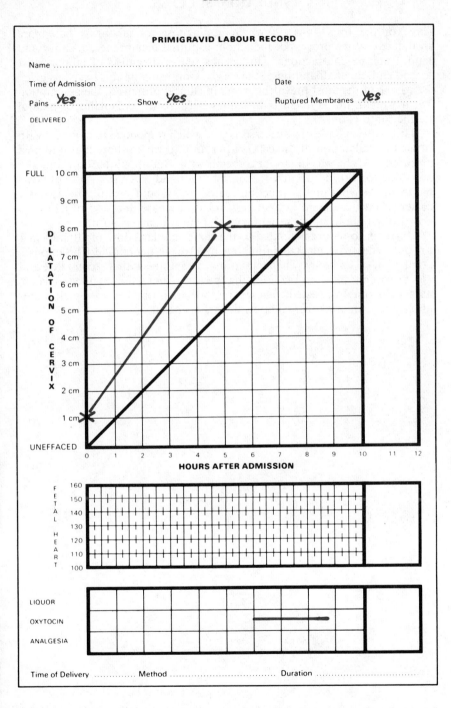

PRIMIGRAVID LABOUR RECORD

Name ....

Time of Admission ....   Date ....

Pains ...*Yes*................   Show ...*Yes*......................   Ruptured Membranes ...*Yes*....

DELIVERED

FULL   10 cm

DILATATION OF CERVIX

9 cm
8 cm
7 cm
6 cm
5 cm
4 cm
3 cm
2 cm
1 cm

UNEFFACED

0   1   2   3   4   5   6   7   8   9   10   11   12

HOURS AFTER ADMISSION

FETAL HEART

160
150
140
130
120
110
100

LIQUOR

OXYTOCIN

ANALGESIA

Time of Delivery ....   Method ....   Duration ....

INDUCTION: SUCCESS

Three of the four signs on which a diagnosis of labour is based are invalidated by the process of induction: ruptured membranes, a 'show' and painful uterine contractions. This means that a diagnosis of labour must depend entirely on dilatation of the cervix. Confusion on this issue has given rise to one of the most prevalent errors in clinical obstetrics: the assumption that a woman on oxytocin is in labour because she complains of painful uterine contractions.

This is an example of a successful case, which responded to oxytocin with progressive dilatation of the cervix after an interval so short that it almost appeared as if she was in labour to begin with. But no matter how long the interval, once 'lift-off' occurred, progress was rapid. Even so it was not possible to say at what point induction ceased and labour began. This is not a matter of great moment in a successful case because duration of labour is recorded as time spent in the delivery unit before a baby is born.

Oxytocin to induce is limited to the same standard dose of 10 units in 1 litre of 5% dextrose, at a maximum rate of 60 drops per minute. This imposes a time limit of six hours. The temptation to continue with a second litre and possibly even a third, in the hope that a caesarean section may be avoided, must be strongly resisted. These are the circumstances in which water intoxication, among other complications, may occur.

GRAPH 25

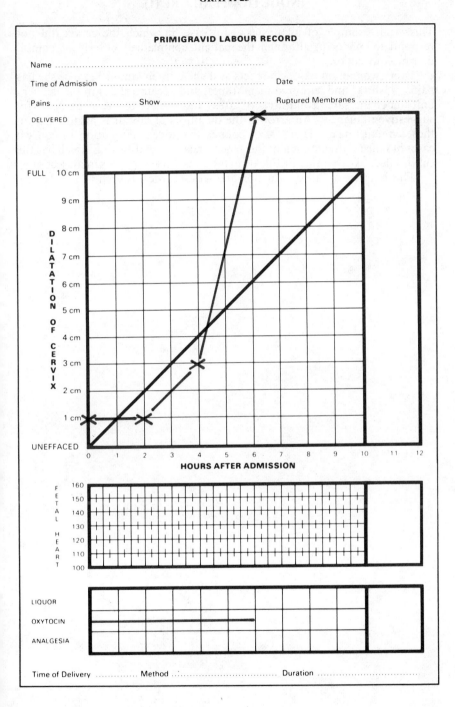

INDUCTION: FAILURE (1)

This is an example of an unsuccessful case, in which the cervix did not respond to oxytocin, although the patient complained bitterly of painful uterine contractions.

Every woman on oxytocin reacts as if she were in labour because she has pains, a 'show' and ruptured membranes, and because she is in the delivery unit under the same conditions of stress and subject to the same powerful suggestive influences. An error in the diagnosis of labour is all too easy in these circumstances. There is, of course, the added temptation to conceal cases of failed induction under the general heading of dystocia, which has the subtle effect of providing justification for an unnecessary caesarean section.

This is a case of failed induction and was recorded as such.

GRAPH 26

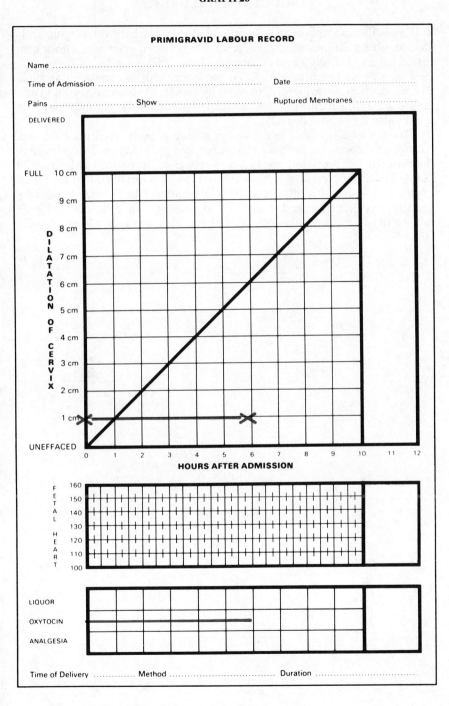

INDUCTION: FAILURE (2)

This is another example of an unsuccessful case, in which the cervix reluctantly yielded, giving the impression that it was being forced open, like a door with rusted hinges. 'Lift-off' never occurred.

This was no less a case of failed induction and was recorded as such. Every induction subsequently delivered by caesarean section is recorded as a failure, because patients are selected for induction on the grounds that they are suitable for vaginal delivery.

There is an alternative to caesarean section in such cases, once the true nature of the condition has been recognized: oxytocin may be discontinued in the reasonable expectation that labour will begin of its own accord within 24 hours. For this reason women should be informed beforehand that the use of oxytocin to induce is not necessarily a commitment to immediate delivery and that oxytocin may be discontinued to await spontaneous labour. Given time, artificial rupture of membranes alone often succeeds where oxytocin fails.

GRAPH 27

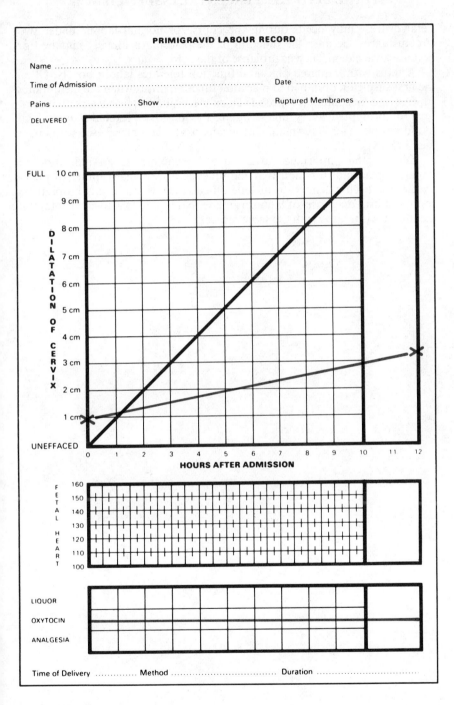

PRIMIGRAVID LABOUR RECORD

Name ....

Time of Admission .... Date ....

Pains .... Show .... Ruptured Membranes ....

DELIVERED

DILATATION OF CERVIX

FULL 10 cm
9 cm
8 cm
7 cm
6 cm
5 cm
4 cm
3 cm
2 cm
1 cm

UNEFFACED

0 1 2 3 4 5 6 7 8 9 10 11 12

HOURS AFTER ADMISSION

FETAL HEART

160
150
140
130
120
110
100

LIQUOR

OXYTOCIN

ANALGESIA

Time of Delivery .... Method .... Duration ....

FETAL DISTRESS: PLACENTAL INSUFFICIENCY

Fetal distress may occur during the course of normal labour under two circumstances: because the function of the placenta is already impaired or because an accident, such as prolapse of the cord, occurs.

A fetus with impaired placental function tolerates labour poorly. Often the first suspicion of impaired placental function arises when the membranes rupture and meconium is released. Thick meconium is regarded as an indication for prompt delivery unless hypoxia is positively excluded by a fetal blood sample. This is the main reason why oxytocin is never used with intact membranes.

Such is the importance attached to meconium as an indication of impaired placental function that the practice of artificial rupture of membranes has been extended to include all cases delivered in this hospital, as soon as a firm diagnosis of labour is made. No liquor at artificial rupture of membranes is treated with the same respect.

GRAPH 28

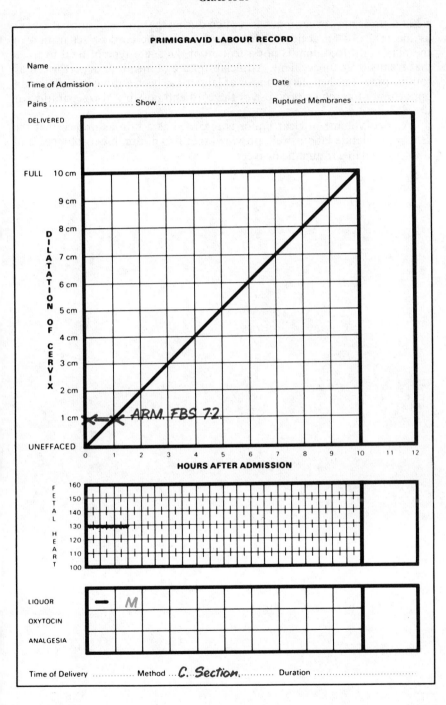

PRIMIGRAVID LABOUR RECORD

Name ....

Time of Admission .... Date ....

Pains .... Show .... Ruptured Membranes ....

DELIVERED

DILATATION OF CERVIX

FULL 10 cm

9 cm

8 cm

7 cm

6 cm

5 cm

4 cm

3 cm

2 cm

1 cm ←— ✕ ARM. FBS 7·2.

UNEFFACED

0 1 2 3 4 5 6 7 8 9 10 11 12

HOURS AFTER ADMISSION

FETAL HEART

160
150
140
130
120
110
100

LIQUOR — M

OXYTOCIN

ANALGESIA

Time of Delivery .... Method ... *C. Section*............ Duration ....

FETAL DISTRESS: ACCIDENT OF LABOUR

Fetal distress may occur much less often during the course of normal labour as the result of an accident: either prolapse of the cord or separation of the placenta. Meconium is not a feature of the acute type of fetal hypoxia that results from an accident. Artificial rupture of membranes performed as routine practice when the diagnosis of labour has been established affords an opportunity to exclude prolapse of the cord and possibly also separation of the placenta.

A good volume of clear liquor is regarded as a firm assurance that the fetus will tolerate labour well, provided that it is not unduly prolonged and does not end in a traumatic delivery.

GRAPH 29

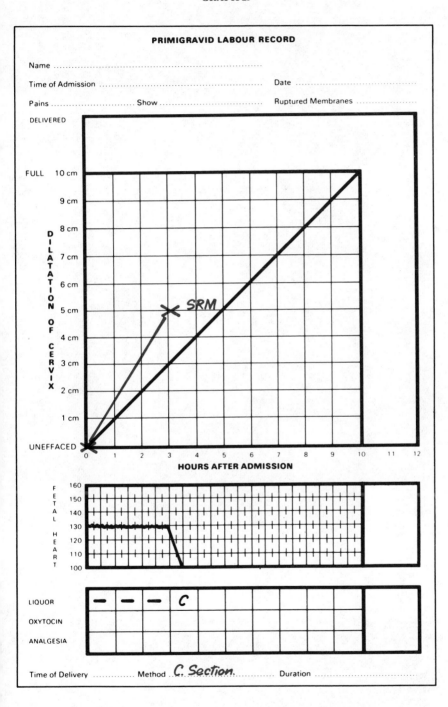

PRIMIGRAVID LABOUR RECORD

Name ....

Time of Admission .... Date ....

Pains .... Show .... Ruptured Membranes ....

DELIVERED

FULL 10 cm

DILATATION OF CERVIX

9 cm
8 cm
7 cm
6 cm
5 cm ✕ SRM
4 cm
3 cm
2 cm
1 cm
UNEFFACED

HOURS AFTER ADMISSION
0 1 2 3 4 5 6 7 8 9 10 11 12

FETAL HEART
160
150
140
130
120
110
100

LIQUOR — — — C

OXYTOCIN

ANALGESIA

Time of Delivery .... Method C. Section .... Duration ....

Multigravid Labour

MULTIGRAVID LABOUR

From the standpoint of labour the multigravid or parous woman may as well belong to a different biological species. Hence the labour record is printed on a different colour paper. Significantly, the sole difference in content is that the word oxytocin is omitted. Lack of appreciation of the reasons for these distinctions leads to the most enduring of all obstetric errors: the practice of extrapolating from a first to a second birth. This results in much unnecessary intervention and iatrogenic disease. There is no basis for comparison as the two events are completely unrelated. The salient features of multigravid labour may be summarized thus.

The duration and consequent stress involved bear no comparison with first labour because the parous woman rarely suffers from inefficient uterine action and because her genital tract has been stretched before. In the event of slow progress, therefore, another explanation should be sought, the most likely being that she is not in labour.

Failure to advance in a parous woman who is in labour is often a manifestation of obstruction arising from a fetal cause. This can be easily overlooked with disastrous consequences because the capacity of the pelvis is taken for granted. The common causes of obstruction are brow presentation and hydrocephalus.

The parous uterus is prone to rupture and this may occur even in the course of normal labour. Oxytocin should be used to stimulate the parous uterus only after most serious consideration and on a strictly individual basis. The diagnosis of labour should be reviewed and the causes of obstruction carefully excluded beforehand.

Epidural anaesthesia has very little application in the parous woman because one in two can expect to be delivered within two hours. In the event of slow progress, epidural anaesthesia is potentially dangerous, because it permits labour to continue, while suppressing evidence of impending rupture. The combination of oxytocin with epidural anaesthesia is particularly dangerous in this regard. Commitment to epidural anaesthesia in a parous woman is based on the false premise that all labours are the same.

GRAPH 30

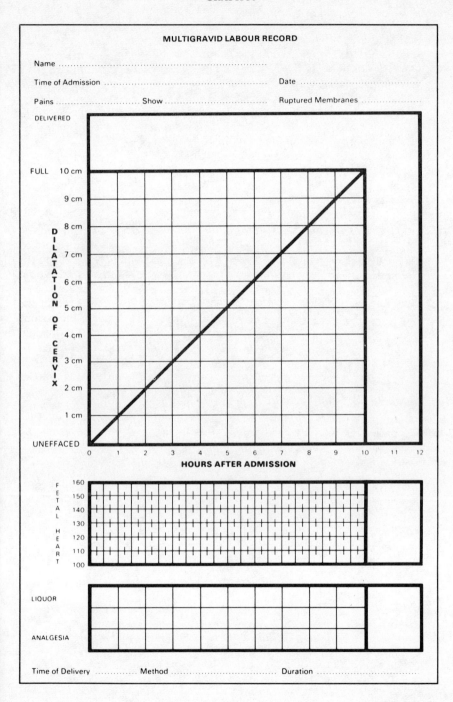

MULTIGRAVID LABOUR RECORD

Name ....

Time of Admission .... Date ....

Pains .... Show .... Ruptured Membranes ....

DELIVERED

FULL   10 cm

9 cm

8 cm

D
I
L   7 cm
A
T   6 cm
A
T   5 cm
I
O   4 cm
N
O   3 cm
F
C   2 cm
E
R   1 cm
V
I
X   UNEFFACED

0   1   2   3   4   5   6   7   8   9   10   11   12

HOURS AFTER ADMISSION

F   160
E   150
T   140
A   130
L   120
H   110
E   100
A
R
T

LIQUOR

ANALGESIA

Time of Delivery .... Method .... Duration ....

SECTION III
Clinical Data

Table 1
National Maternity Hospital—Comparative figures for 20 years

Year	1965	1970	1975	1976	1977	1978	1979	1980	1981	1982	1983	1984
Babies born	5063	6255	7430	7553	7590	8101	8450	8849	8964	8653	8159	7853
Perinatal deaths	185	180	157	122	150	143	132	126	109	98	107	94
Necropsies	181	180	157	121	148	141	132	122	109	97	104	91
Mortality rate	36.5	28.8	21.1	16.2	19.8	17.6	15.6	14.2	12.2	11.3	13.1	12.0
Caesarean section (%)	4.2	4.2	4.1	3.7	4.4	4.7	5.5	4.9	5.5	5.2	6.0	4.2
Induction (%)	28.5	36.0	14.7	12.3	8.8	9.4	12.1	13.4	8.2	10.0	13.4	10.8
Forceps (%)	12.2	7.7	11.0	9.5	9.2	5.7	4.4	6.5	7.0	6.2	6.6	6.3

COMPARATIVE FIGURES FOR 20 YEARS

This table requires little in the way of explanation. As the general principle that underlies the practice of this hospital is to achieve the best results with the least interference, attention is directed to the following items:

Mortality rate

Perinatal mortality still represents the best objective measure of standards of practice in terms of the child. Notice is drawn to the exceptional number of post-mortem examinations performed. This has special relevance to trauma; death is all too easily attributed to hypoxia, without post-mortem examination.

Caesarean section

In terms of the mother, caesarean section rates serve the same function. The incidence of caesarean section was low and remained so throughout the entire period. These figures stand in sharp contrast with levels of 10 or even 20% in similar institutions elsewhere.

Induction

The incidence of induction increased to 36% in 1970. Thereafter there was an abrupt decline when a selective, instead of a statistical, approach to poorly defined risk factors, mainly pre-eclampsia and post-maturity, was adopted.

Forceps

For ease of comparison with other centres, the incidence of forceps is expressed here as a percentage of total births, whereas in practice some 90% of forceps were performed in primigravidae. With the introduction of Active Management of Labour as the standard procedure, the incidence of forceps declined to 6%, subsequently to rise again, partly, at least, due to the use of epidural anaesthesia, albeit on a limited scale.

Table 2
National Maternity Hospital—Analysis of hospital population*

Year	1965	1970	1975	1976	1977	1978	1979	1980	1981	1982	1983	1984
Maternal age												
<20	3	6	8	7	7	7	6	6	6	6	6	6
20–29	50	58	61	62	62	61	61	60	61	60	61	60
30–39	39	31	27	28	28	30	31	32	31	32	31	32
40+	8	5	4	3	3	2	2	2	3	2	2	2
Parity												
1	26	33	38	36	35	35	35	35	35	35	35	36
2, 3, 4	51	51	52	54	55	55	56	55	56	56	56	55
5+	23	16	10	10	10	10	9	10	9	9	9	9
Birth-weight												
2.5 kg or less	7	6	4	4	4	5	5	3	4	3	3	4
Socioeconomic group												
1, 2	33	34	34	33	35	34	38	45	46	48	42	46
3	26	26	34	36	35	35	36	29	27	25	28	22
4, 5	41	40	32	31	30	31	26	26	27	27	30	32

*Socioeconomic factors expressed to the nearest per cent.

ANALYSIS OF HOSPITAL POPULATION

A progressive reduction in the perinatal mortality rate of some 66% over these 20 years was associated with notable changes in the social background of the population served. There can be little doubt that these changes contributed more to the improvement in this respect than any advance in medical science. The chief items are listed in Table 2.

Maternal age

Maternal age has an important bearing on perinatal mortality; thus our experience has been of a two-fold increase after 35 years. The percentage of mothers aged 35 years or more fell by one-half—from 25 to 11—during this time.

Parity

A similar change was evident in the pattern of fertility. The percentage of grande multiparae declined by more than one-half—from 23 to 9—with a corresponding increase in first births.

Birth-weight

A striking improvement occurred under this heading, where a reduction by one-half, to the low level of 4%, could not but have a profound effect on results, especially on the component of perinatal mortality represented by neonatal death where, congenital malformation apart, birth-weight is the main issue.

Socioeconomic group

This hospital caters for a representative cross-section of the community. Although not so accurately defined as age and parity, there seemed to be a substantial reduction in the percentage of mothers in the semi-skilled and unskilled groups. This change in the nature of employment seemed to correspond with an obvious improvement in living standards all round.

Table 3
National Maternity Hospital—Clinical circumstances of perinatal deaths

Year	1965	1970	1975	1976	1977	1978	1979	1980	1981	1982	1983	1984
Total births	5063	6255	7430	7553	7590	8101	8450	8849	8946	8653	8159	7853
Dead when referred	22	16	8	3	3	5	3	4	1	1	2	2
Died before labour	43	56	70	50	55	40	55	57	57	37	58	39
Died in labour ward	16	24	8	7	20	11	11	10	5	5	11	8
Neonatal deaths	47	40	38	30	33	32	24	20	16	21	9	5
Congenital malformations	57	44	33	32	39	55	39	35	30	34	27	40
Total deaths	185	180	157	122	150	143	132	126	109	98	107	94

CLINICAL CIRCUMSTANCES OF PERINATAL DEATHS

This table places the perinatal deaths in the clinical context in which they occurred. There were considerable improvements under all headings except one: Died before labour.

By way of contrast, the reductions elsewhere are the more striking, because they occurred against the background of an increase of more than 50% in total births.

Dead when referred

The virtual elimination of this category of death reflects the trend to combined antenatal care and eventual hospital delivery, which took place at a national level during these years; this item accounts for a reduction of 4 per 1000 in the overall perinatal mortality rate.

Died before labour

This category includes late fetal deaths that occurred before the onset of labour. Most were unexplained, but intrauterine growth retardation was a common finding.

Improvement under this heading accounts for 4 per 1000 in the perinatal mortality rate.

Died in labour ward

Apropos the management of labour, which is the subject of this manual, the improvement here represents a reduction of 2 per 1000 in the perinatal mortality rate.

Neonatal deaths

This category accounts for a reduction of 9 per 1000 in the perinatal mortality rate, which should be considered in the light of the decline in the incidence of low birth-weight referred to in Table 2.

Congenital malformations

The reduction under this heading, which accounts for 6 per 1000 in the perinatal mortality rate, raises questions that are outside the scope of the present text.

Table 4
National Maternity Hospital—Rupture of the uterus

Year	1965	1970	1975	1976	1977	1978	1979	1980	1981	1982	1983	1984	Total*
Cases	4	8	4	5	4	5	6	3	5	3	2	2	84
Primigravidae	0	0	0	0	0	0	0	0	0	0	0	0	0

*The figures for 1966–9 and 1971–4 are incorporated in the totals, although they are otherwise not included in the table.

RUPTURE OF THE UTERUS

This is the ultimate expression of serious injury to the mother.

There was no case of rupture of the uterus in almost 50 000 consecutive primigravidae delivered in the largest maternity hospital in the British Isles, during a period of 20 years—despite the fact that oxytocin was used in some 15 000 to ensure efficient uterine action during labour—and without regard to the possibility of cephalopelvic disproportion.

Dehiscence of a caesarean section scar accounted for 51 of the 84 cases of rupture of the uterus in multigravidae.

The confidence necessary to use oxytocin effectively derives ultimately from the information contained in this and the following table.

Table 5
National Maternity Hospital—Traumatic intracranial haemorrhage in first-born infants

Year	1965	1970	1975	1976	1977	1978	1979	1980	1981	1982	1983	1984	Total*
Births	1327	2054	2778	2675	2606	2803	2897	3106	3107	2960	2885	2812	47979
TICH	6	2	4	0	1	1	1	0	2	2	0	1	34
Breech	2	1	3	0	0	0	0	0	0	1	0	0	15
Vertex	4	1	1	0	1	1	1	0	2	1	0	1†	19
Forceps	4	1	1	0	1	1	1	0	2	1	0	0	18

*The figures for 1966–9 and 1971–4 are incorporated in the totals, although they are otherwise not included in the table.
†This exception was a thanatophoric dwarf.

TRAUMATIC INTRACRANIAL HAEMORRHAGE IN FIRST-BORN INFANTS

This is the ultimate expression of serious injury to the child.

There were 34 cases of traumatic intracranial haemorrhage in first-born infants: 19 cephalic and 15 breech presentations. All but 1 of the 19 cases of traumatic intracranial haemorrhage in first-born infants with cephalic presentations were delivered with forceps. Traumatic intracranial haemorrhage occurred once in association with spontaneous delivery in almost 50 000 firstborn infants—and this despite the fact that oxytocin was used in some 15 000 to ensure efficient uterine action, without regard to the possibility of cephalopelvic disproportion.

This should be read in conjunction with the previous table.

Table 6
National Maternity Hospital—Cerebral dysfunction in mature infants

Year	1970	1975	1976	1977	1978	1979	1980	1981	1982	1983	1984	Total*
Babies born	6255	7430	7553	7590	8101	8450	8849	8964	8653	8159	7853	117183
Cerebral dysfunction	17	25	8	6	21	18	29	32	17	22	9	267
Hypoxia	12	17	4	3	21	15	23	30	17	22	7	210
Accident of labour	3	5	3	0	0	2	1	0	0	0	0	26
Trauma	0	0	0	0	0	0	1	0	0	0	1	9
Other causes	2	3	1	3	0	1	4	2	0	0	1	22

*The figures for 1971–4 are incorporated in the totals, although they are otherwise not included in the table.

CEREBRAL DYSFUNCTION IN MATURE INFANTS

Permanent brain damage that could have been avoided may well be regarded as the ultimate failure in obstetric practice.

So that these may be known and kept under surveillance, all cases of cerebral dysfunction identified in the course of routine examination for this purpose by our neonatologists are placed on record.

Cerebral dysfunction is defined as a state of abnormal muscle tone or altered primitive reflexes, which occurs in term infants who weigh 2500 g or more. Preterm infants born before 37 completed weeks and infants of low birth-weight are specifically excluded.

Hypoxia is clearly the most important factor in this regard, and typically this was the penultimate stage in a process that had existed before labour began: placental insufficiency, in other words. Accidents of labour cover prolapse of the cord and abruption of the placenta. Among the cases of trauma, there were six forceps and three breech deliveries. Other causes include drugs, infections and metabolic disorders.

Table 7
National Maternity Hospital—Diagnosis of labour

Pains	890
'Show'	586
Spontaneous rupture of membranes	269

DIAGNOSIS OF LABOUR

This table lists the evidence with which 1000 consecutive primigravidae presented at the delivery unit of this hospital in the belief that labour had started.

Clearly some 10% were mistaken, because they failed to pass the initial test of painful uterine contractions. A very high proportion of those who passed this test had the additional evidence of a 'show' or spontaneous rupture of membranes. Notice was taken of a 'show' only when this appeared before the membranes ruptured.

Some with painful uterine contractions had neither of these two signs, in which case the crucial decision as to whether or not to retain was based entirely on complete effacement of the cervix.

Table 8
National Maternity Hospital—Duration
of labour in primigravidae

Hours	Percentage
< 2	12
2–4	26
4–6	28
6–8	20
8–10	9
10–12	3
12 +	2
	100

DURATION OF LABOUR IN PRIMIGRAVIDAE

Duration of labour is synonymous with time spent in the delivery unit of this hospital before the baby is born: all cases are included, whether or not a state of labour existed—a point of special significance in induction.

The mean duration of labour in primigravidae, without treatment, is somewhat less than six hours.

The composite figures given opposite are, like those in the next table, based on two series, each of 1000 consecutive primigravidae, five years apart; treated cases are included.

Table 9
National Maternity Hospital—Dilatation
at admission in primigravidae

	Percentage
Not effaced	7
Effaced	54
2, 3 cm	24
4, 5 cm	4
6, 7 cm	3
8, 9 cm	3
Full dilatation	5
	100

DILATATION AT ADMISSION IN PRIMIGRAVIDAE

Effacement of the cervix refers to the length of the canal, from above downwards.

Dilatation of the cervix refers to the external os only, when effacement is complete.

The cervix is not effaced in some 7% and is already fully dilated in some 5% of primigravidae admitted to this hospital in labour. These two extremes do not relate well with time spent in labour at home.

Many authors adopt the simple device of excluding those cases at the lower levels of dilatation and in doing so exclude the problem cases, both in diagnosis and treatment.

The multigravid cervix is an entirely different organ.

Table 10
National Maternity Hospital–Obstetrical
norms in primigravidae

	Percentage
Caesarean section	5
Induction	10
Forceps	10
Epidural	5
Acceleration	30

Kielland's forceps or ventouse are not used.

OBSTETRICAL NORMS IN PRIMIGRAVIDAE

A paradoxical feature of contemporary practice is a steady increase, almost everywhere, in the rate of medical—or more important, surgical—intervention, despite a remarkable improvement in general health and a precipitous fall in perinatal mortality. There is, indeed, a widespread tendency to attribute these improved results to this very intervention. Table 1 shows how false this assumption can be; this table suggests that obstetricians might be better advised simply to hold the line as results continue to improve. Certainly, above anything else, iatrogenic disease—whether physical or emotional—must be avoided.

In conclusion, therefore, and based largely on experience recounted here, certain norms have been adopted to ensure that the rising tide of intervention is kept in check. The figures for multigravidae are lower—generally much lower—under each heading.

List of Publications

1. O'Driscoll K. (1966) Rupture of the uterus. *Proceedings of the Royal Society of Medicine* 59: 65.
2. O'Driscoll K., Jackson R.J.A. & Gallagher J.T. (1969) Prevention of prolonged labour. *British Medical Journal* ii: 477–480.
3. O'Driscoll K., Jackson R.J.A. & Gallagher J.T. (1970) Active management of labour and cephalopelvic disproportion. *British Journal of Obstetrics and Gynaecology* 77: 385–389.
4. O'Driscoll K. (1972) Impact of active management on delivery unit practice. *Proceedings of the Royal Society of Medicine* 65: 697–698.
5. O'Driscoll K., Stronge J.M. & Minogue M. (1973) Active management of labour. *British Medical Journal* iii: 135–137.
6. O'Driscoll K. (1975) An obstetrician's view of pain. *British Journal of Anaesthesia* 47: 1053–1059.
7. O'Driscoll K. & Stronge J.M. (1975) Active management of labour and occipito-posterior position. *Australian and New Zealand Journal of Obstetrics and Gynaecology* 15: 1–4.
8. O'Driscoll K. & Stronge J.M. (1975) The active management of labour. *Clinics in Obstetrics and Gynaecology* 2: 3–17.
9. O'Driscoll K., Carroll C.J. & Coughlan M. (1975) Selective induction of labour. *British Medical Journal* iv: 727–729.
10. Boylan P. (1976) Oxytocin and neonatal jaundice. *British Medical Journal* ii: 564–465.
11. O'Driscoll K., Coughlan M., Fenton V. & Skelly M. (1977) Active management of labour: care of the fetus. *British Medical Journal* ii: 1451–1453.
12. O'Driscoll K., Meagher D., MacDonald D. & Geoghegan F. (1981) Traumatic intracranial haemorrhage in firstborn infants and delivery with obstetric forceps. *British Journal of Obstetrics and Gynaecology* 88: 577–581.
13. O'Driscoll K. & Foley M. (1983) Correlation of decrease in perinatal mortality and increase in cesarean section rates. *Obstetrics and Gynecology* 61: 1–5.
14. Boylan P. & O'Driscoll K. (1983) Improvement in perinatal mortality rate attributed to spontaneous preterm labor without use of tocolytic agents. *American Journal of Obstetrics and Gynecology* 145: 781–783.
15. O'Driscoll K., Foley, M. & MacDonald D. (1984) Active management of labor as an alternative to caesarean section for dystocia. *Obstetrics and Gynecology* 63: 485–490.
16. MacDonald D., Grant A., Sheridan-Pereira M., Boylan P. & Chalmers I. (1985) The Dublin randomized controlled trial of intrapartum fetal heart rate monitoring. *American Journal of Obstetrics and Gynecology* 152: 524–539.
17. Garcia J., Corry M., MacDonald D., Elbourne D. & Grant A. (1985) Mothers' views of continuous electronic fetal heart monitoring and intermittent auscultation in a randomised controlled trial. *Birth* 12: 79–85.

Index